C000112191

QUICK-FIX FAT LOSS

by Joe Warner and Jon Lipsey

Art Editor Ian Ferguson
Managing Editor Chris Miller
Photography Glen Burrows
Model Daniel Ventura
Additional Photography iStock

Publisher Steven O'Hara
Publishing Director Dan Savage
Marketing Manager Charlotte Park
Commercial Director Nigel Hole

Printed by William Gibbons and Sons, Wolverhampton

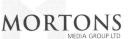
MEDIA GROUP LTD

Published by Mortons Media Group Ltd,
Media Centre, Morton Way,
Horncastle, LN9 6JR
01507 529529

To license this product please contact Carlotta Serantoni on +44 (0) 20 79076550 or email carlotta_serantoni@dennis.co.uk
To syndicate content from this product please contact Ryan Chambers on +44(0) 20 7907 6132 or email Ryan_Chambers@dennis.co.uk

Contents

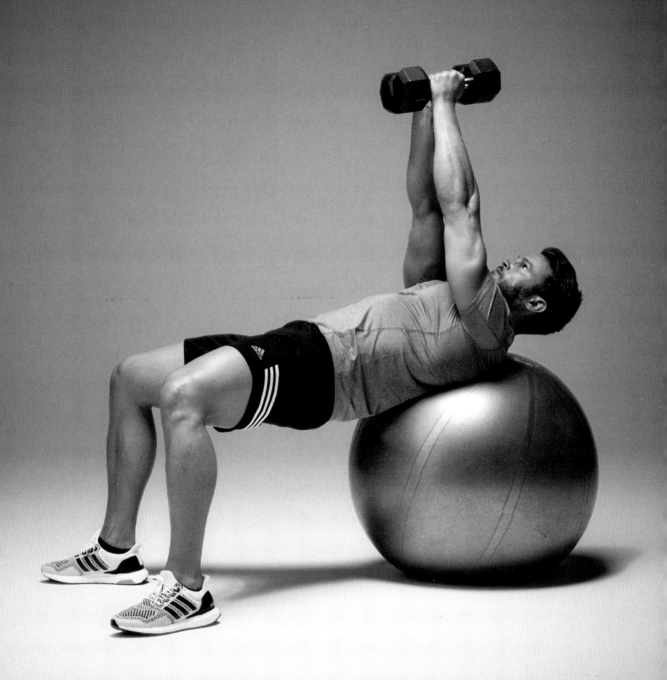

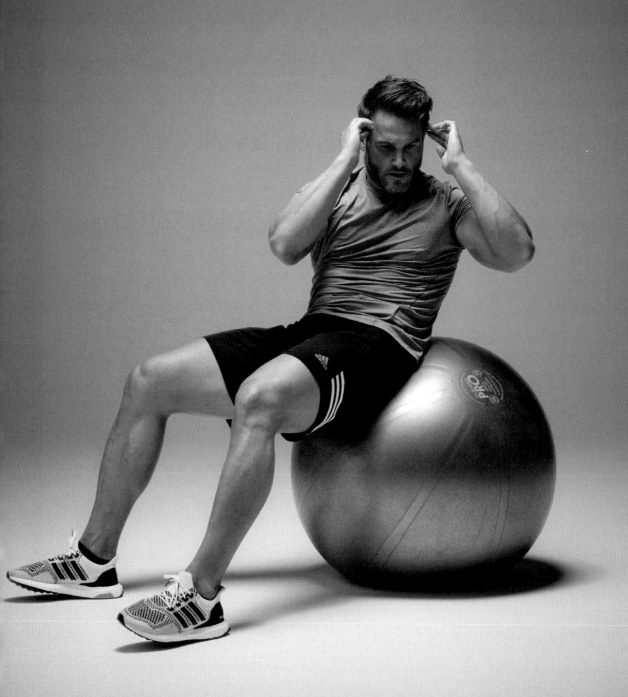

Welcome!

Welcome to your new eight-week training and eating plan that will help you shift body fat fast and allow you to build the body you've always wanted. In many ways you've already done the hardest part of any fat loss journey: you've bought this book and proved you are ready to make a commitment to improve your health and build a leaner, fitter body.

That doesn't mean stripping away body fat is easy – if it was, we'd all be walking around looking like underwear models. But this book reveals how you can improve your body in the easiest way possible – through a challenging training plan and a sensible, sustainable nutrition approach. Once you know the best ways to eat and exercise, you will shed your unwanted fat sooner than you thought possible.

So take some time to read about how our eight-week fat-torching plan works, then put the advice into action. You'll be amazed how quickly your body changes shape.

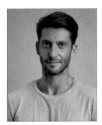

Joe Warner Editor
@JoeWarnerUK

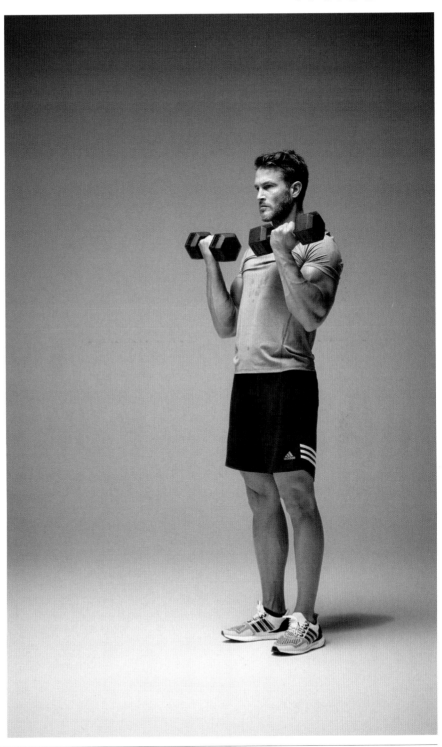

Get lean in just eight weeks

Have you tried to lose fat in the past to build a fitter, healthier and leaner body? Most of us have, but most of us would also admit that we ultimately failed to make the desired changes we wanted. Even if you did have some success, the chances are that you have put back on some of that lost weight.

But you now hold in your hands the only guide you need to building a better body for life. Using our eight-week training plan, which has four workouts a week, will help you shift body fat fast

– and help you keep it off by giving you all the training knowledge you need to turn your body into a fat-burning machine every time you exercise.

At the same time, you'll get a physical upgrade by adding lean muscle mass across your chest, shoulders, back, arms and legs. What's more, the diet plan in the book will give you a flexible, nutritious (and delicious) guide to eating for better health as well as fat loss, enabling you to build a leaner body and reveal hard abs.

Five things you need to do before you begin

1 The first thing you need to do is read through the eight-week workout plan (p16) and familiarise yourself with how the sessions work so you start the plan fully informed and confident you know what you do to get results.

2 Then turn to the exercise form guide chapter and ensure that you know how to perform each move perfectly to work your muscles in the most effective way to burn fat and build muscle. This section starts on p118.

3 Make every session more effective with a workout notebook. Ahead of each workout, write down the plan, then tick off the sets as you complete them. Note the weights you've lifted to ensure you keep progressing.

4 Clean out your cupboards to bin the foods you know you need to avoid in the pursuit of burning body fat as quickly as possible. Then fill your fridge with more of the foods you do need. Turn to p96 for more details.

5 Make a playlist of motivational music. Exercising to your favourite tunes makes hard training feel easier, and listening to the tracks you love can also alleviate stress. Turn to p14 for some more quick workout tips.

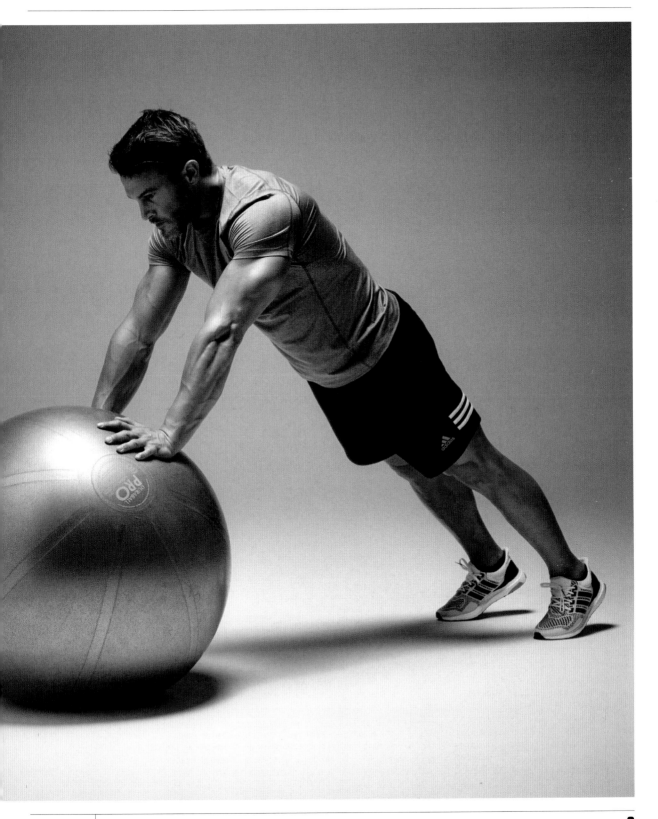

YOUR 8-WEEK QUICK-FIX FAT LOSS PLAN

When you're trying to reduce the amount of body fat you're carrying – especially that fat that gets stored around your middle – it can be tempting to dramatically reduce the amount of food you eat (especially carbs) and dramatically increase the amount of exercise you do (especially in the form of long and slow running).

But that's a trap you don't want to fall into. Blitzing your belly in the most effective way possible means taking a smarter approach to both eating and exercising. That's where this eight-week workout programme comes in. It will place the perfect stimulus on your body to encourage it to tap into its fat stores to use as fuel.

It will also add lean muscle mass to your major muscle groups – specifically your shoulders, chest, back, arms and legs. Although building more muscle mass might seem a lower priority than losing your belly right now, adding more muscle will help make a huge difference to how you look with your shirt off. Ultimately you'll radically transform your physique into a lean, mean, fit and healthy machine.

By following this training plan you'll get leaner and more defined, as well as stronger and more mobile. You'll also gain more training confidence and experience, which will enable you to take on more advanced training approaches once you've lost that spare tyre around your midriff and want a new training goal to work towards.

This eight-week plan involves four circuit workouts a week. Circuits are sessions where you do one set of an exercise, then move on to the next exercise without resting. You only rest once you've completed a round of all the exercises listed. This is effective because the lack of rest forces both your muscles and your cardio system to work overtime to keep your body moving, and it's these exertions that torch body fat for fuel and instruct your body to grow your muscles back bigger and stronger.

The circuits here comprise bodyweight exercises and dumbbell moves that raise your heart rate and keep it high while working a large number of muscle groups in every session, an approach that turns your body into a fat-burning furnace. Not only do you torch more calories during your workout, but you also burn more calories in the hours and days after a session as your body recovers from your lung-busting, muscle-taxing exertions. Yes, the sessions are tough, but you'll feel great as soon as they're over – and that's what it takes to transform your body for the better in just eight weeks.

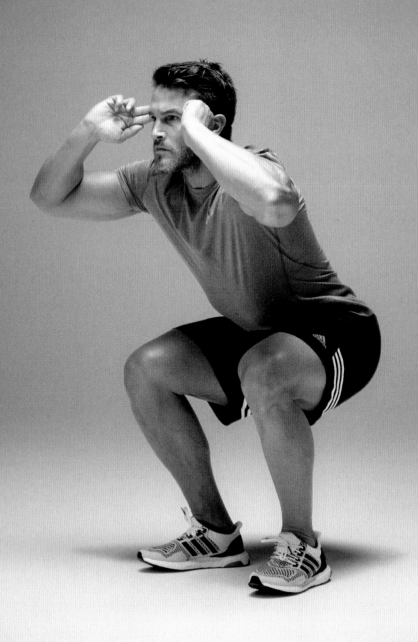

How to make every workout your best ever

Follow these six tips to get the fat loss results you want faster

 Make time for your training

Every Sunday spend 10 minutes booking the week's training sessions into your work diary. If you have them down in black and white and give them the same importance as your professional commitments, you will treat them as such and never use an excuse to skip a session. The most important element when trying to make significant improvements to your body is consistency – the more consistent you can be with your training, the faster you'll burn fat.

 Start to keep a workout diary

Recording your progress is a fantastic way to stay on top of your fat loss challenge. After every training session, write down the weights you lifted for each exercise – next time you do that move, aim to go slightly heavier to ensure you're progressing. You can also record other data such as energy levels, motivation levels, hours of sleep and other important lifestyle factors, giving you a detailed record of how you feel as well as how you look. You'll know at a glance if you're improving, and get an idea of what to change if not.

 Take a weekly progress pic

A great way to track your progress and stay motivated is to take weekly pictures of your body. Seeing how your body changes for the better week by week can be extremely inspiring and keep you focused on moving closer to your goal. Just make sure you take the photo on the same day each week at the same time – ideally in the same place and with the same lighting – to give you the most accurate image of how you're doing.

 Enlist some social support

Another highly effectively means of getting – and staying – motivated is to enlist the support of friends and family. Tell your close circle about your fat loss goal and why you are undertaking a programme to achieve it. If they know what you're doing and why, it will help in many ways, especially when you're finding it hard to keep going. It'll also make them less likely to twist your arm to do things that will harm your chances of success.

 Get a friend involved

Even better than getting support from your friends is signing up one or more of them to get into better shape with you. Numerous scientific studies have indicated that training with someone else increases the motivation to train in the first place, and that you also work out harder and more efficiently than when you do it alone. A little bit of friendly competition can be the extra spur you need to train harder and eat better to strip away fat.

 Reward all your hard work

If you have previously struggled with motivation levels then you can deploy some simple tactics to make this attempt more successful. One could be to put aside some money every time you complete a workout. It might not seem much, but the simple act of doing so gives you a reason to train, and the cash will soon add up – and eventually go some way towards the new wardrobe of slim-fit T-shirts you're going to need.

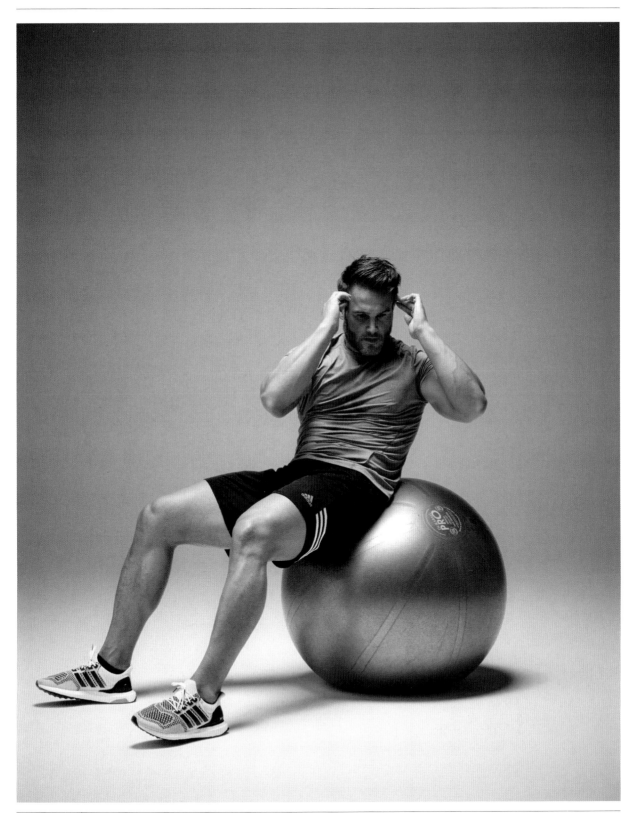

How it works
Here's the theory behind the plan

HOW DOES THE PLAN WORK?
This eight-week workout plan will add muscle while stripping away fat because it's a progressive programme that pushes you a little further outside of your comfort zone every time you train. This approach gives your body no choice but to keep adapting to the increasingly difficult challenges. Always asking your body to work a bit harder is tough, and there'll be times you want to quit, but every session you successfully complete will take you a step closer to a better body.

DO I NEED TO FOLLOW IT EXACTLY?
If you want to get the best results possible you need to follow it to the letter. The plan has been designed to push your body hard, with four workouts every week, and chopping and changing will reduce its effectiveness. Consistency is crucial to any successful fat loss attempt so you need to make sure you do each of the four weekly sessions for the full eight weeks, even if that means sacrificing some of your free time. It will be worth it in the end.

WHAT WEIGHT DO I LIFT?
Many of the moves in this programme are bodyweight moves, but some require the use of dumbbells to provide more resistance. Finding your starting weight for these exercises may need a little trial and error, and it's best to start light if in doubt, then increase the weight in subsequent sets and subsequent sessions. If you finish the final couple of circuits and feel like you could have done a few more reps of the dumbbell moves, the weight is too light.

WHAT DO I DO AFTER THE PLAN?
The beauty of following this eight-week plan is that you'll gain muscle size and strength as well as new muscle while you strip away fat. This will leave you in shape to take your training to the next level once you've completed it. You could focus on some strength or hypertrophy training, or you can simply repeat this plan, but your new strength means you'll be able to start with heavier weights and keep progressing accordingly.

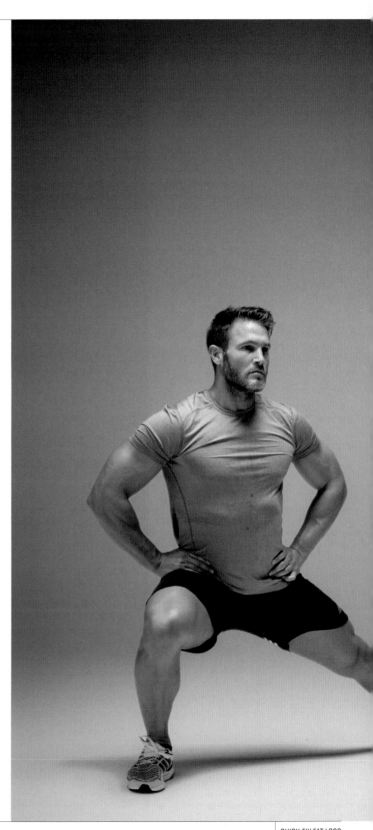

14

Key workout variables

Here's what the main training terms mean in practice

EXERCISE

The selection of exercises you perform in a given session is one of the most important workout variables because these determine which muscles you work and how much training time you give to a particular muscle group. All the workouts in this eight-week plan are made up of six exercises, which you'll perform in a circuit (see next column). For most of this programme the first four moves you do in each circuit alternate between lower-body and upper-body exercises. This is a proven approach to keep your heart rate high – which helps burn fat – as it is forced to pump blood back and forth between your torso and legs. The final two moves per circuit target your abs.

CIRCUITS

Every one of the four weekly sessions you'll be doing over eight weeks is a circuit made up of six different exercises. Each circuit lists the moves in order. You start with move 1 and perform it for the stated length of time (see next column). Once that time is up, you go straight into the second exercise without stopping to rest, then repeat this pattern for the rest of the exercises. You rest only after you've completed all six moves. The number of circuits you do in each workout changes from week to week so that you keep your body out of its comfort zone, which is one of the quickest and most effective ways to reduce your body-fat levels.

TIME

Instead of counting the number of reps of each exercise you have to do before you can move on to the next, every workout in this plan is based on doing each of the six moves for a set amount of time – either 30, 45 or 60 seconds. This approach means you can focus on performing each exercise properly (sticking to the comprehensive form guides beginning on p118) rather than trying to rush through a rep count, which will make your form suffer and results hard to come by. Focusing on quality movement patterns to work your heart, lungs and muscles harder is the best way to force your body to give up its fat stores for fuel to shed body fat as quickly as possible.

REST

The length of time you rest between exercises and circuits has a huge impact on your fat loss progress. Most importantly, rest breaks should not be too long because that gives your heart, lungs and muscles enough recovery time so that they are never truly pushed out of their comfort zone, making impressive physique changes hard to achieve. In this eight-week plan, though, you never rest between the exercises of a circuit – you only get to have a breather at the end of each circuit, and that will be for as little as two minutes and no more than three. It's essential you stick to these limits if you want to burn fat fast.

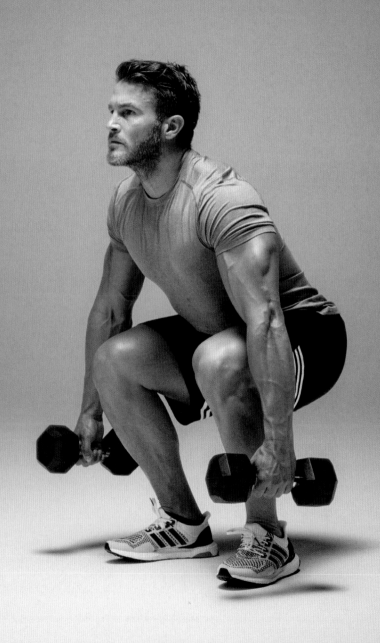

WEEK 1

The first week of your eight-week plan is designed to get your muscles moving properly so you can start burning fat and building muscle right away. You'll do each move for 30 seconds, then move on to the next exercise. Only rest once you've completed the sixth and final exercise of each circuit, and limit your rest to two minutes to make your workouts as effective as possible. Good luck!

Workout 1

This bodyweight circuit will get your heart pumping hard and fast

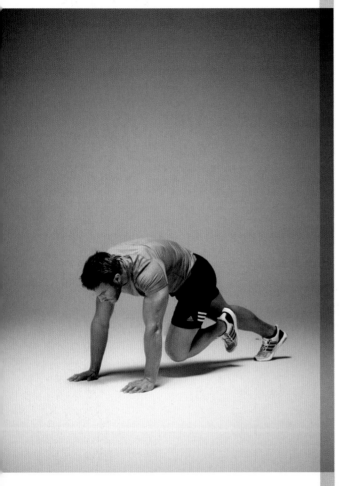

Complete

4

circuits in total

1 Squat

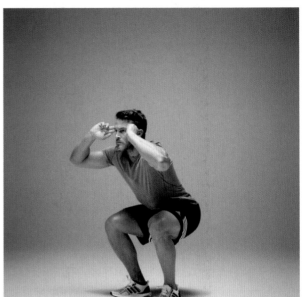

TIME 30sec   **FORM** p141

2 Press-up

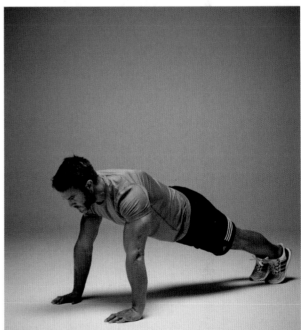

TIME 30sec   **FORM** p157

3 Lunge

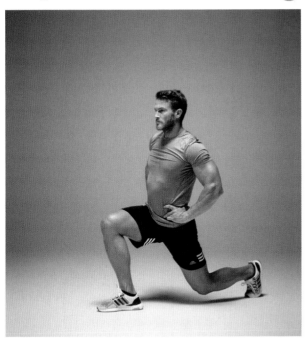

TIME 30sec   FORM p131

4 Mountain climber

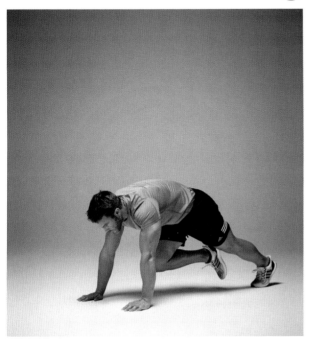

TIME 30sec   FORM p155

5 Crunch

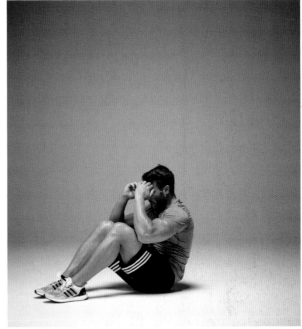

TIME 30sec   FORM p121

6 Reverse crunch

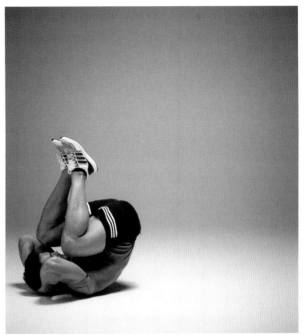

TIME 30sec REST 2min   FORM p158

Workout **2**

A bodyweight circuit that works all your major muscle groups

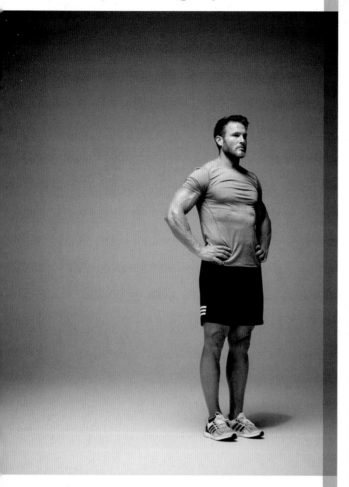

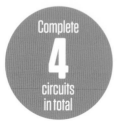

Complete
4
circuits
in total

1 Split squat

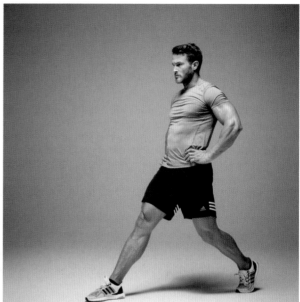

TIME 30sec   FORM p140

2 Wide press-up

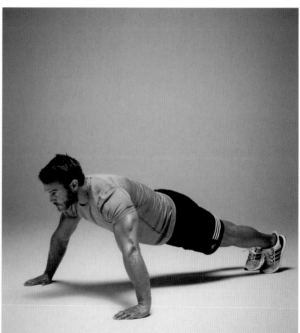

TIME 30sec   FORM p162

3 Side lunge

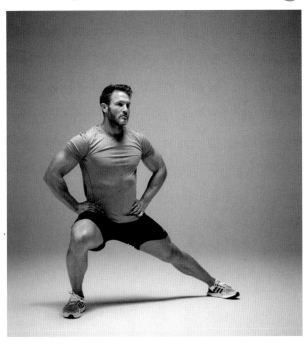

TIME 30sec   **FORM** p139

5 Bicycle

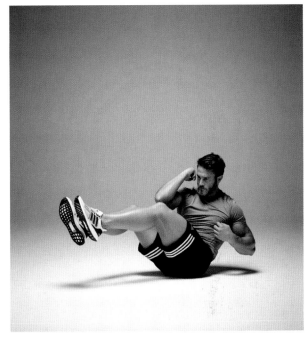

TIME 30sec   **FORM** p120

4 Diamond press-up

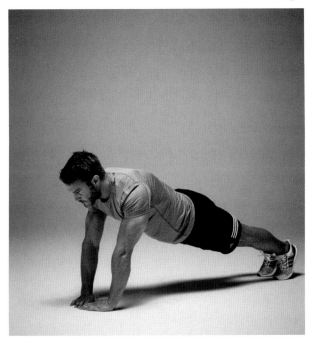

TIME 30sec   **FORM** p123

6 Plank

TIME 30sec **REST** 2min   **FORM** p156

Workout 3

The addition of dumbbells as extra resistance works you far harder

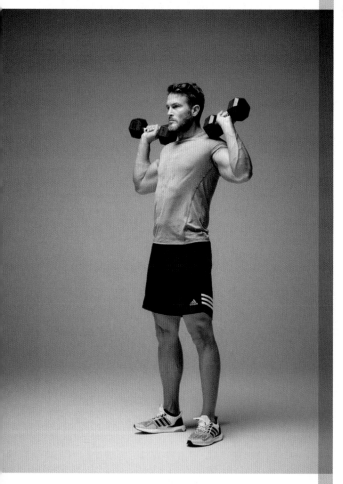

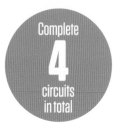

Complete

4

circuits
in total

1 Dumbbell squat

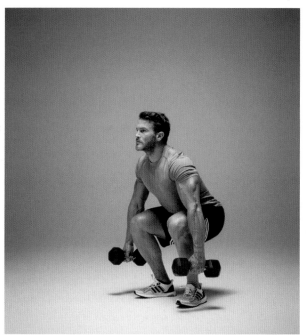

TIME 30sec   FORM p141

2 Dumbbell bent-over row

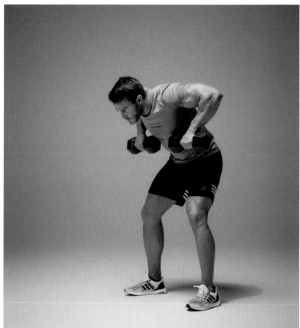

TIME 30sec   FORM p125

3 Dumbbell lunge

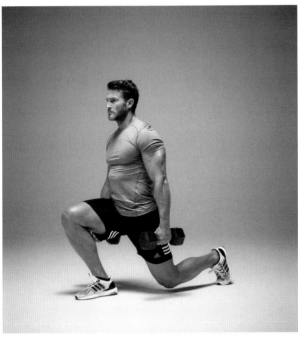

TIME 30sec   **FORM** p131

5 Leg raise

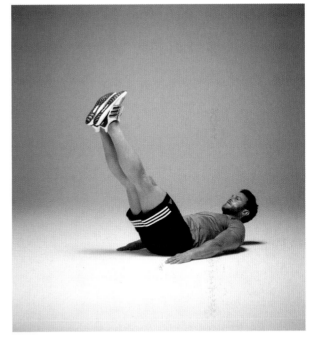

TIME 30sec   **FORM** p154

4 Dumbbell shoulder press

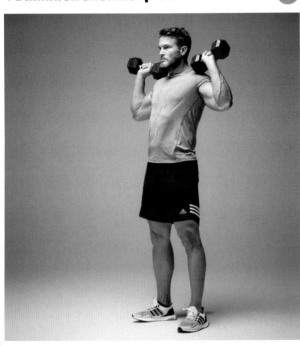

TIME 30sec   **FORM** p138

6 Plank

TIME 30sec **REST** 2min   **FORM** p156

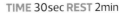

Workout **4**

It's the final circuit of the week, so push yourself as hard as you can

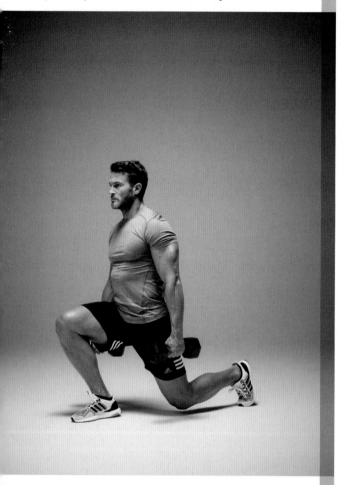

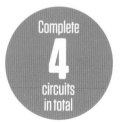

Complete

4

circuits
in total

1 Dumbbell split squat

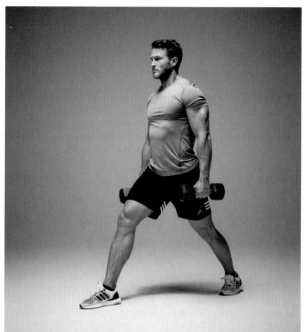

TIME 30sec   FORM p140

2 Dumbbell biceps curl

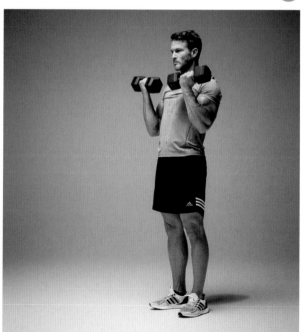

TIME 30sec   FORM p126

3 Dumbbell side lunge

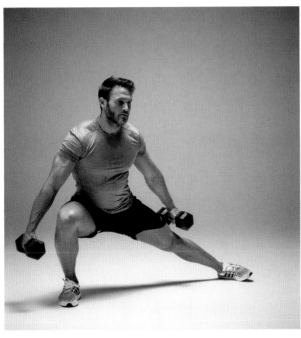

TIME 30sec
FORM p139

5 V-sit

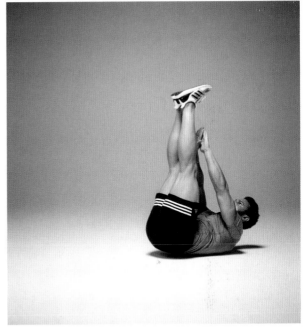

TIME 30sec
FORM p161

4 Dumbbell triceps kick-back

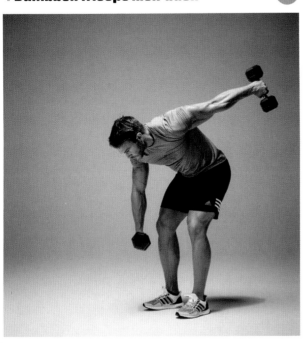

TIME 30sec
FORM p143

6 Side plank

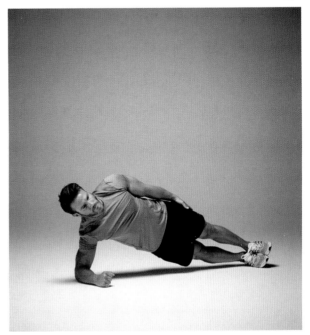

TIME 30sec REST 2min
FORM p159

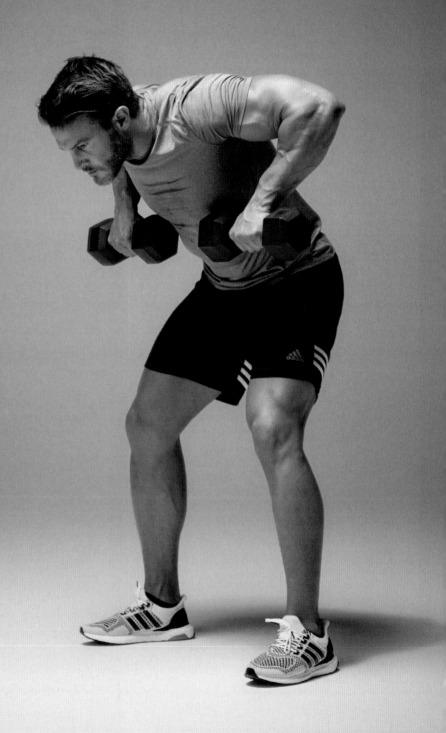

WEEK 2

The four circuits this week are the same as in week 1 but with a big difference that'll make your heart, lungs and muscles work even harder: you'll do each move for 45 seconds, up from 30 seconds in the previous week. This is a significant increase in workload, so you'll get an extra minute to rest between circuits.

Workout 5

Focus on moving through a full range of motion for every rep

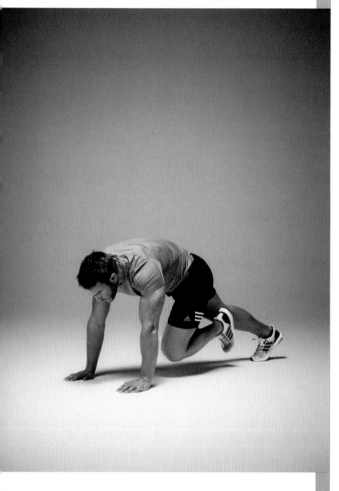

Complete
4
circuits
in total

1 Squat

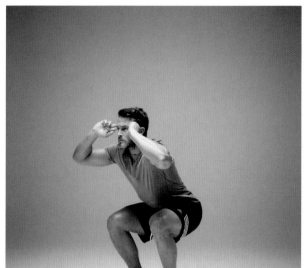

TIME 45sec　　　　　　　　　FORM p141

2 Press-up

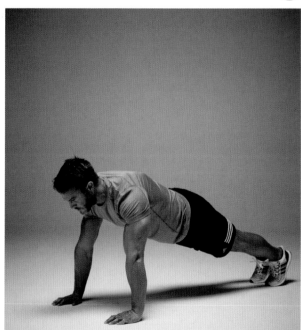

TIME 45sec　　　　　　　　　FORM p157

3 Lunge

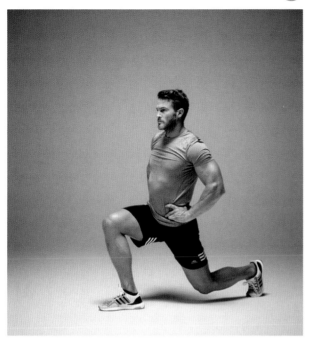

TIME 45sec   FORM p131

4 Mountain climber

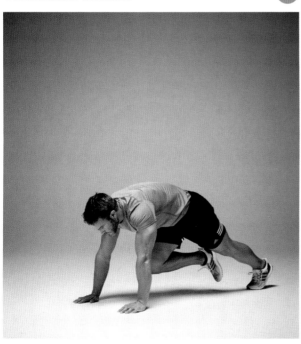

TIME 45sec   FORM p155

5 Crunch

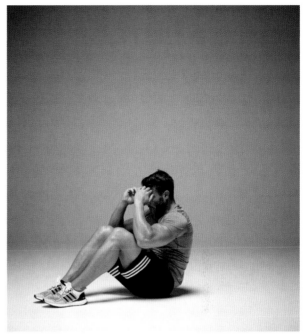

TIME 45sec   FORM p121

6 Reverse crunch

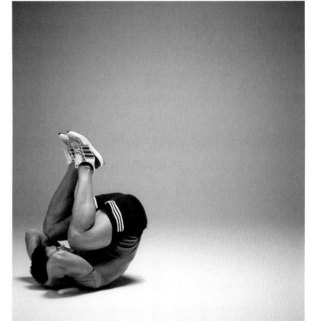

TIME 45sec REST 3min   FORM p158

Workout **6**

Make sure you stick to the three-minute rest periods

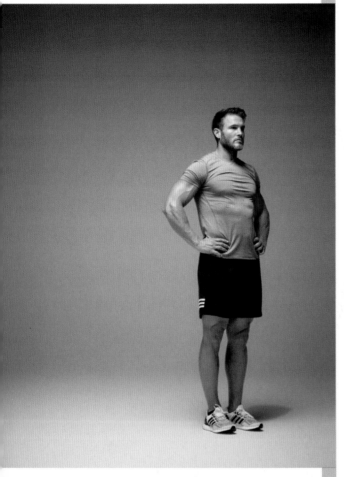

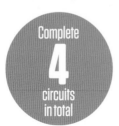

Complete
4
circuits
in total

1 Split squat

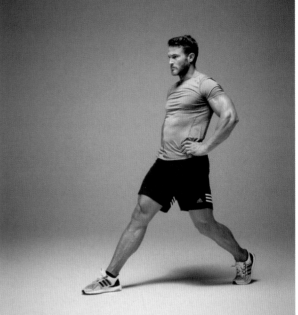

TIME 45sec

FORM p140

2 Wide press-up

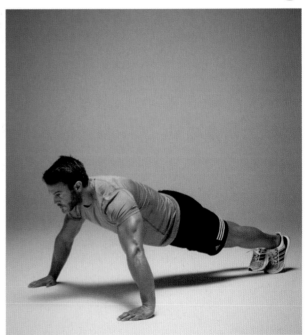

TIME 45sec

FORM p162

3 Side lunge

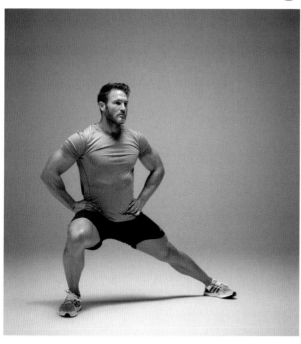

TIME 45sec   **FORM** p139

5 Bicycle

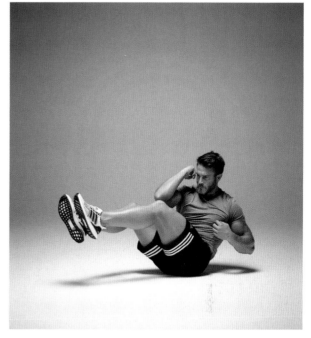

TIME 45sec   **FORM** p120

4 Diamond press-up

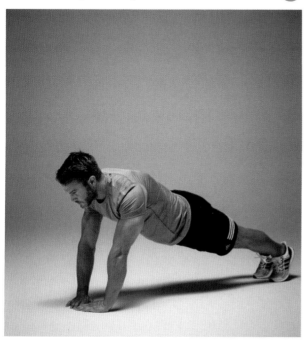

TIME 45sec   **FORM** p123

6 Plank

TIME 45sec **REST** 3min   **FORM** p156

Workout 7

If the reps are too easy, then switch to heavier dumbbells

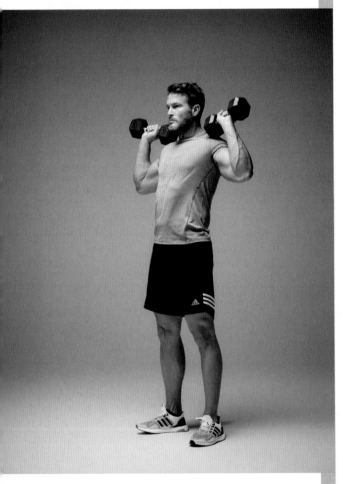

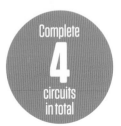

Complete
4
circuits
in total

1 Dumbbell squat

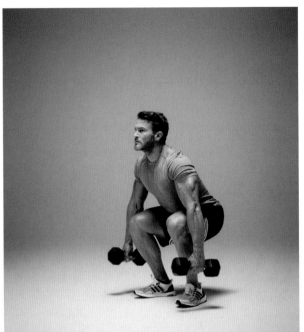

TIME 45sec

FORM p141

2 Dumbbell bent-over row

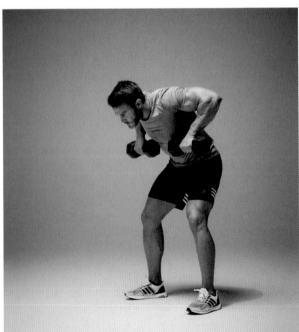

TIME 45sec

FORM p125

3 Dumbbell lunge

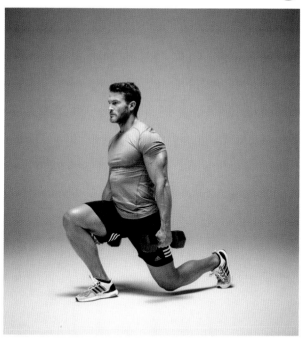

TIME 45sec   FORM p131

4 Dumbbell shoulder press

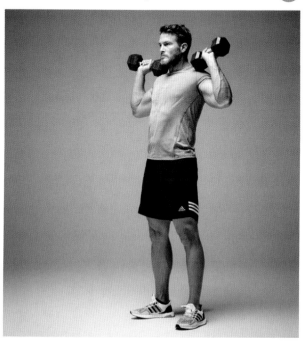

TIME 45sec   FORM p138

5 Leg raise

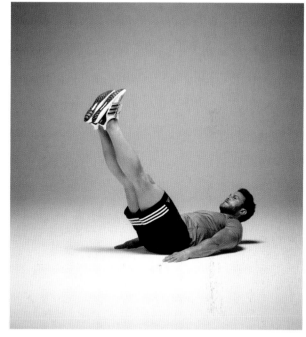

TIME 45sec   FORM p154

6 Plank

TIME 45sec REST 3min   FORM p156

Workout **8**

If you start to struggle switch to
lighter dumbbells and keep going

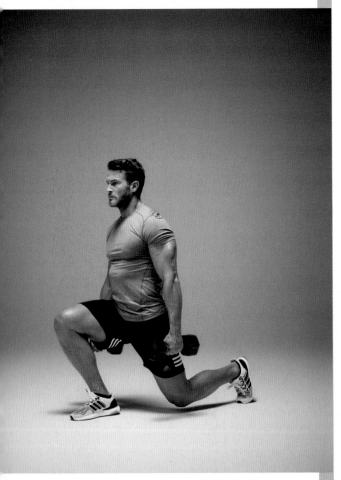

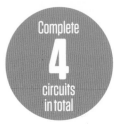

Complete

4

circuits
in total

1 Dumbbell split squat

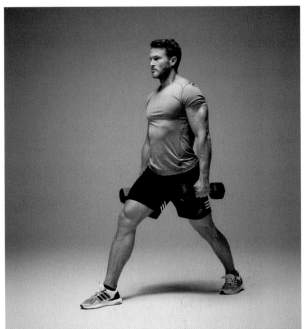

TIME 45sec   **FORM** p140

2 Dumbbell biceps curl

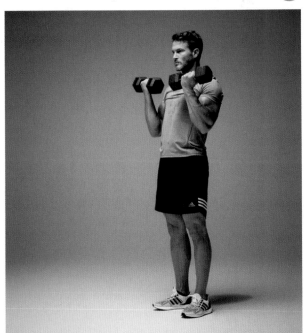

TIME 45sec   **FORM** p126

3 Dumbbell side lunge

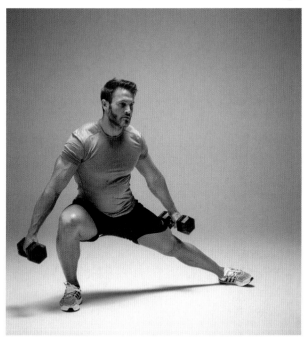

TIME 45sec   **FORM** p139

5 V-sit

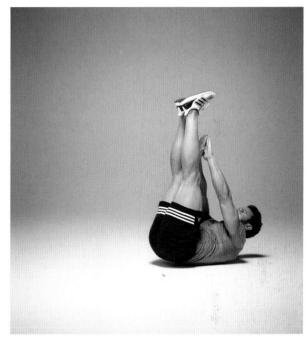

TIME 45sec   **FORM** p161

4 Dumbbell triceps kick-back

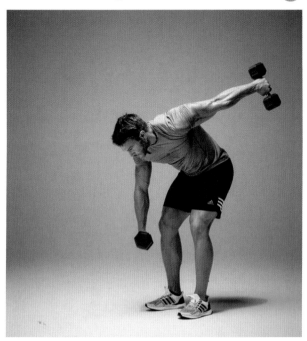

TIME 45sec   **FORM** p143

6 Side plank

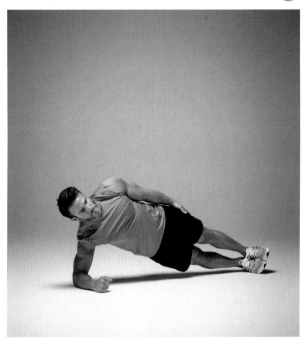

TIME 45sec **REST** 3min   **FORM** p159

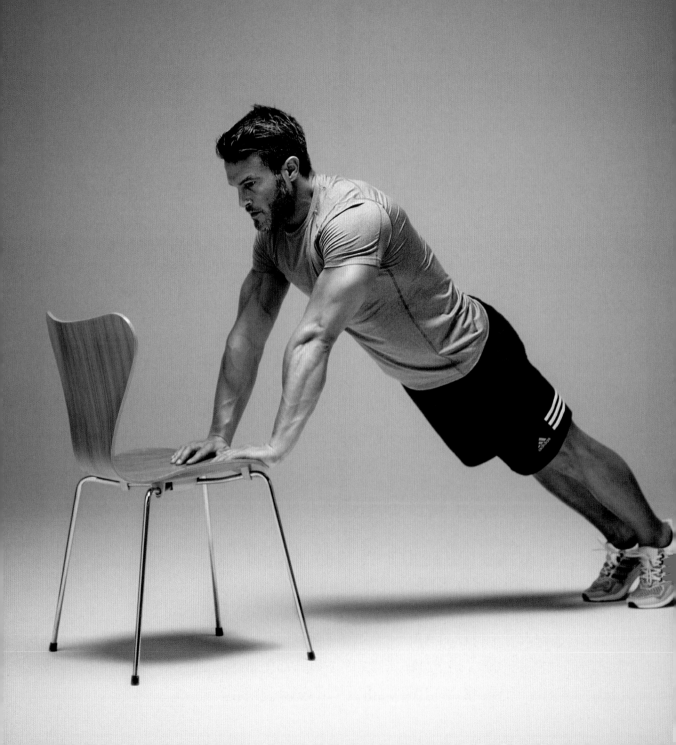

WEEK 3

You're already a quarter of the way through the plan, and it's time to change the workouts so that you keep your body out of its comfort zone by forcing it to guess what's coming next. The moves are different and while there's still four circuits, you'll do each move for 45 seconds but take only two minutes of rest between circuits.

Workout **9**

Do each move for 45 seconds and rest for two minutes at the end

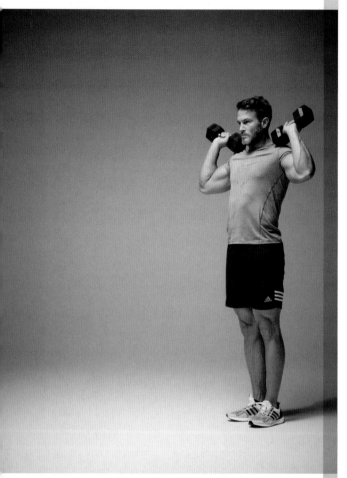

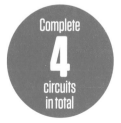

Complete
4
circuits
in total

1 Dumbbell lunge press

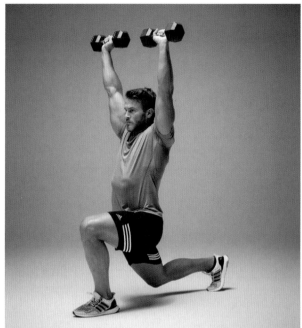

TIME 45sec   **FORM** p133

2 Incline press-up

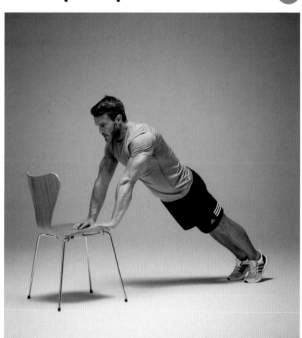

TIME 45sec   **FORM** p153

3 Dumbbell lunge curl

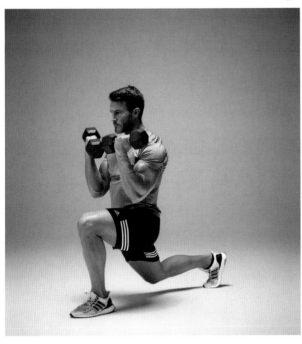

TIME 45sec   **FORM** p132

5 Dumbbell crunch

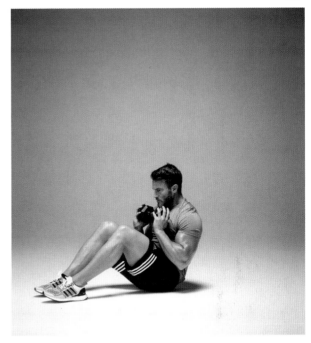

TIME 45sec   **FORM** p127

4 Decline press-up

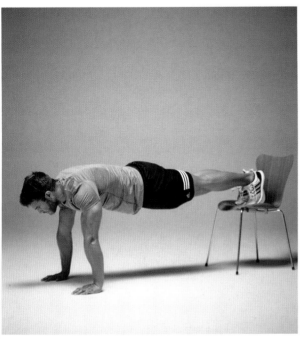

TIME 45sec   **FORM** p148

6 Reverse crunch

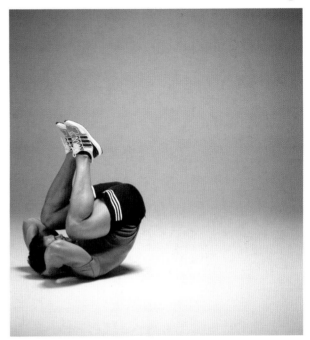

TIME 45sec **REST** 2min   **FORM** p158

Workout 10

Perform each rep of each move quickly but with correct form

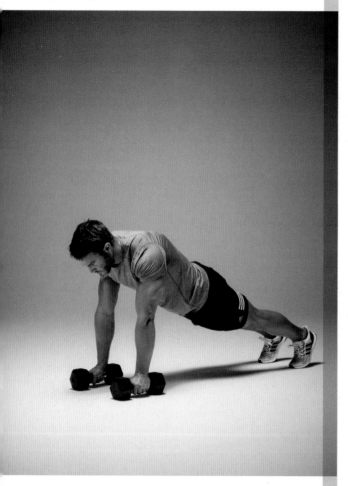

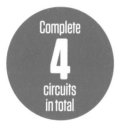

Complete
4
circuits
in total

1 Dumbbell squat curl

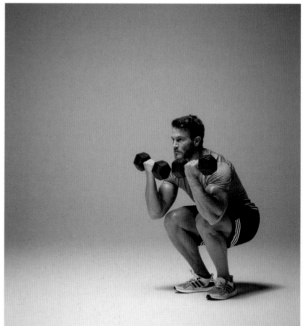

TIME 45sec   **FORM** p142

2 Dumbbell bent-over row

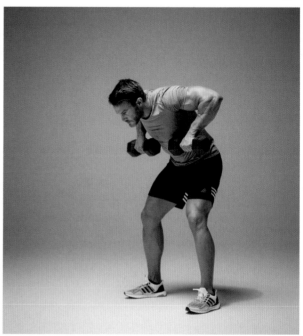

TIME 45sec   **FORM** p125

3 Dumbbell squat

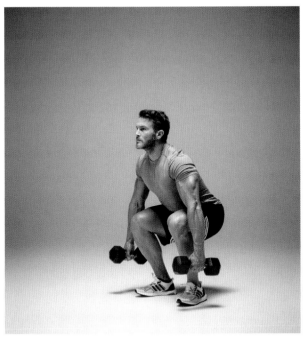

TIME 45sec   FORM p141

4 Dumbbell renegade row

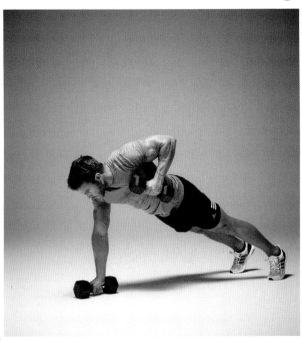

TIME 45sec   FORM p135

5 Leg raise

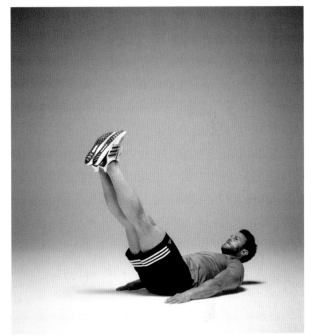

TIME 45sec   FORM p154

6 Plank

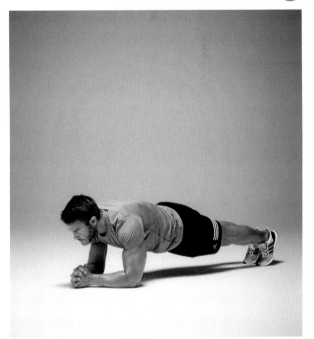

TIME 45sec REST 2min   FORM p156

Workout 11

Attempt to keep your core tight for the duration of each circuit

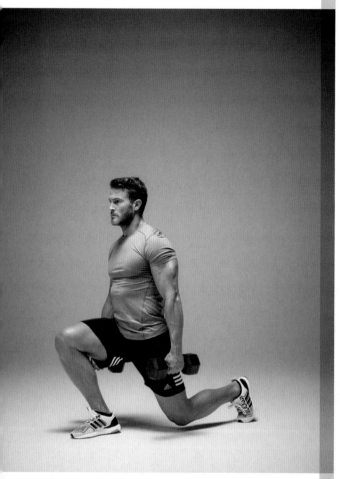

Complete

4

circuits in total

1 Dumbbell split squat

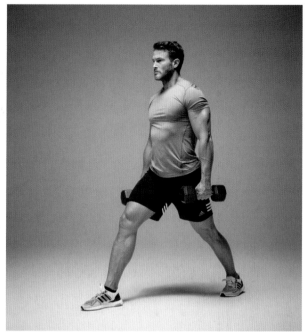

TIME 45sec   FORM p140

2 Dumbbell front raise

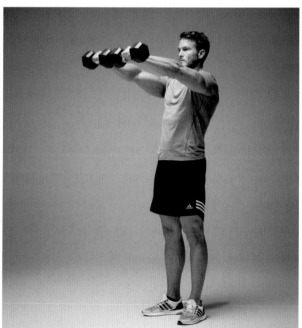

TIME 45sec   FORM p128

3 Dumbbell side lunge

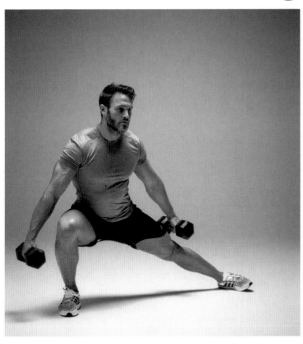

TIME 45sec   FORM p139

4 Dumbbell lateral raise

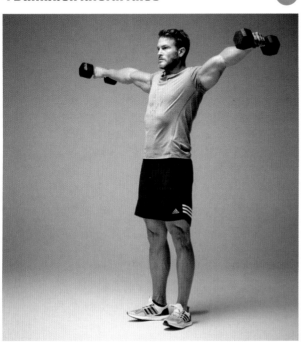

TIME 45sec   FORM p130

5 Mountain climber

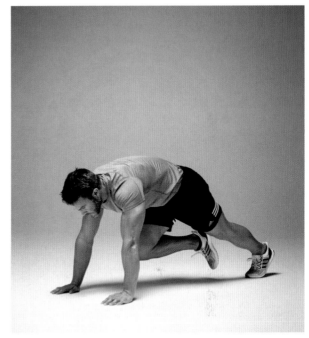

TIME 45sec   FORM p155

6 Plank

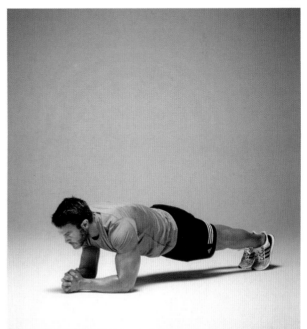

TIME 45sec REST 2min   FORM p156

Workout 12

Focus on breathing deeply and consistently to take in more air

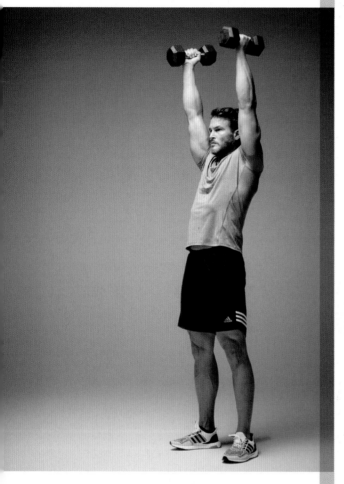

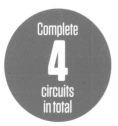
Complete
4
circuits
in total

1 Dumbbell squat

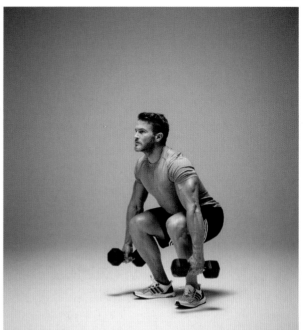

TIME 45sec   **FORM** p141

2 Dumbbell hammer press

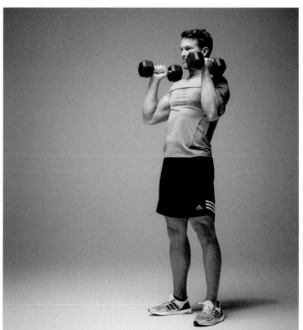

TIME 45sec   **FORM** p129

3 Dumbbell lunge

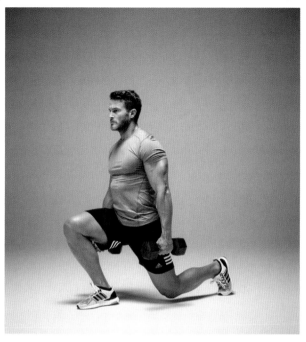

TIME 45sec   FORM p131

4 Dumbbell triceps extension

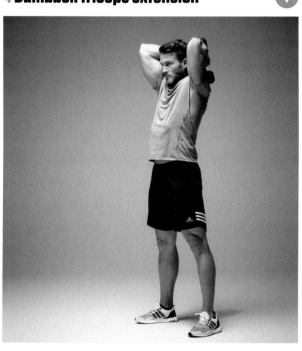

TIME 45sec   FORM p144

5 V-sit

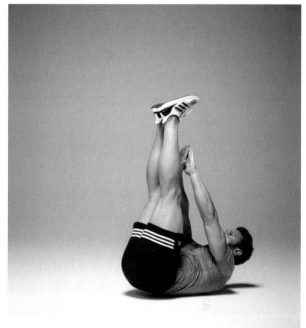

TIME 45sec   FORM p161

6 Side plank

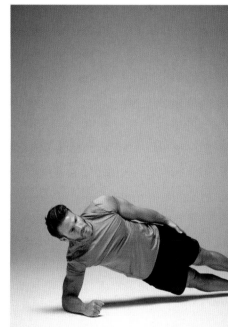

TIME 45sec REST 2min   FORM p159

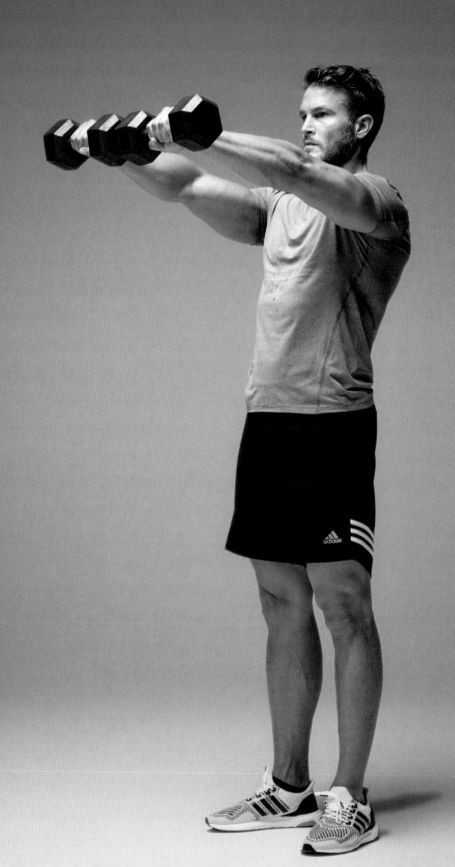

WEEK 4

To ensure you're burning away body fat as quickly as possible – while also placing the right stimulus on your muscles to force them to grow bigger and stronger – this week's workout moves are in the same order as week 3, but now you'll do each exercise for a full minute. You also get three minutes to recover between circuits.

Workout **13**

Do each move for 60 seconds and rest for three minutes at the end

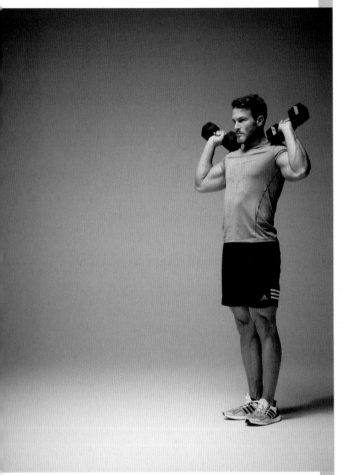

Complete
4
circuits
in total

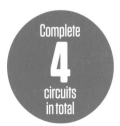

1 Dumbbell lunge press

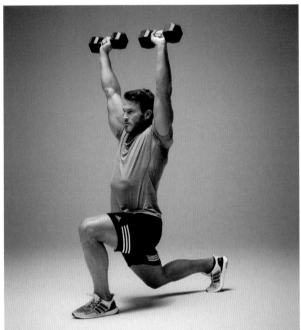

TIME 60sec · **FORM** p133

2 Incline press-up

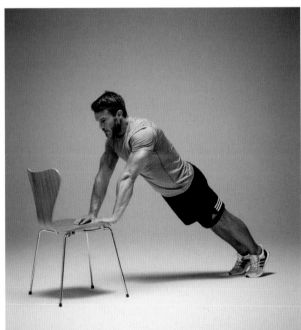

TIME 60sec · **FORM** p153

3 Dumbbell lunge curl

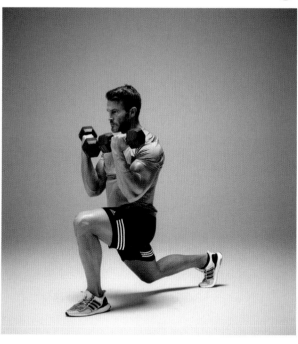

TIME 60sec

FORM p132

4 Decline press-up

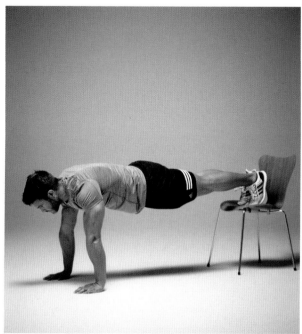

TIME 60sec

FORM p148

5 Dumbbell crunch

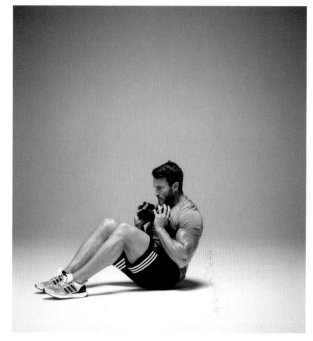

TIME 60sec

FORM p127

6 Reverse crunch

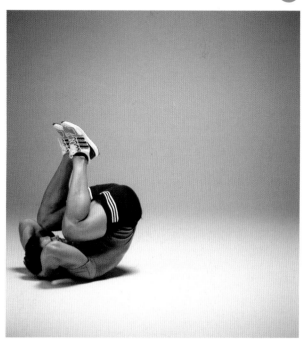

TIME 60sec **TIME** 3min

FORM p158

Workout 14

Don't be afraid to use heavier weights if the moves feel too easy

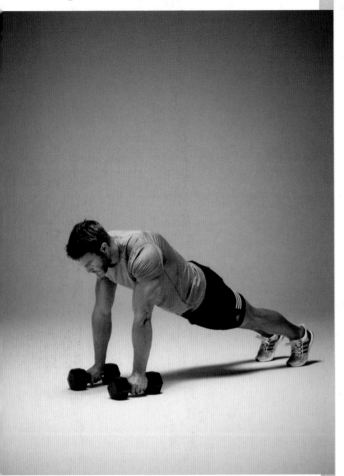

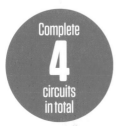

Complete **4** circuits in total

1 Dumbbell squat curl

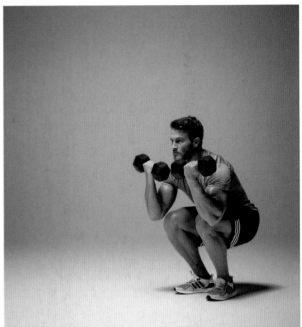

TIME 60sec   **FORM** p142

2 Dumbbell bent-over row

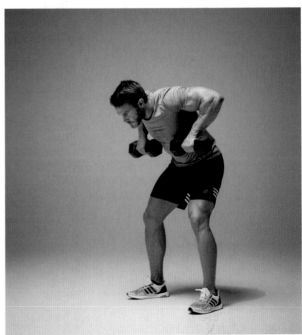

TIME 60sec   **FORM** p125

3 Dumbbell squat

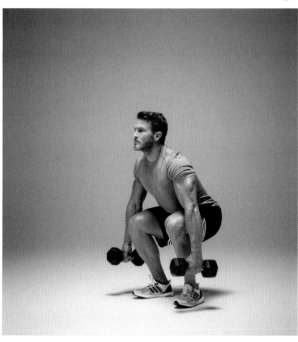

TIME 60sec   **FORM** p141

5 Leg raise

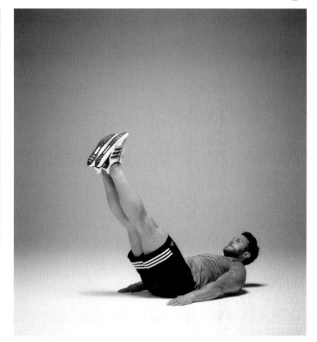

TIME 60sec   **FORM** p154

4 Dumbbell renegade row

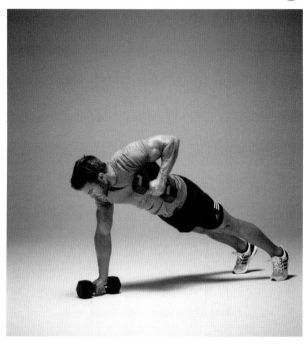

TIME 60sec   **FORM** p135

6 Plank

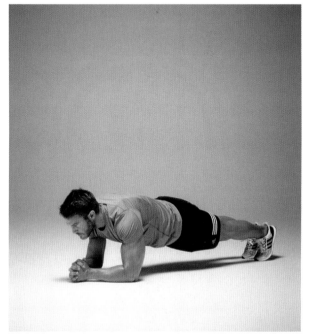

TIME 60sec **REST** 3min   **FORM** p156

Workout **15**

Move your muscles through
their full range for every rep

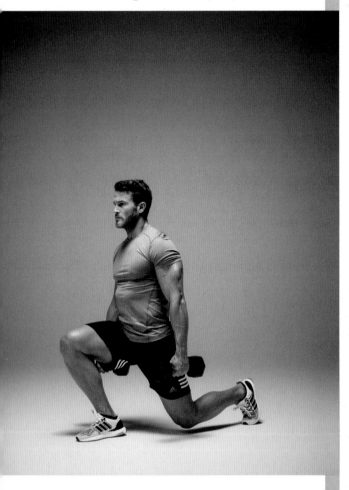

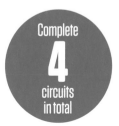

Complete
4
circuits
in total

1 Dumbbell split squat

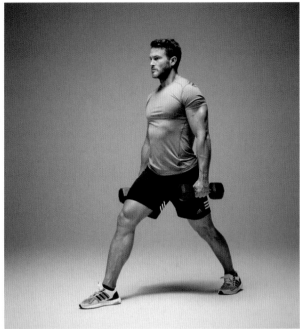

TIME 60sec   **FORM** p140

2 Dumbbell front raise

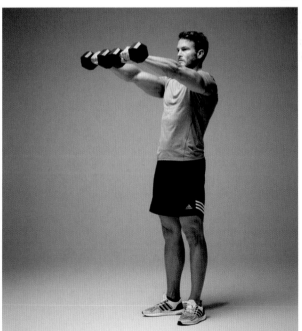

TIME 60sec   **FORM** p128

3 Dumbbell side lunge

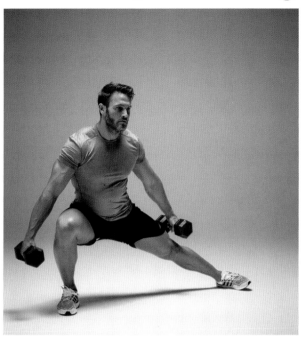

TIME 60sec **FORM** p139

5 Mountain climber

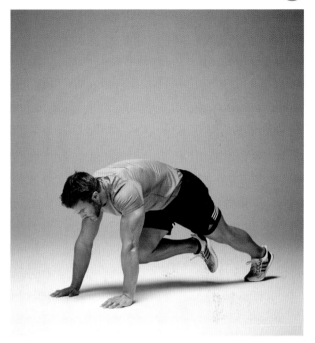

TIME 60sec **FORM** p155

4 Dumbbell lateral raise

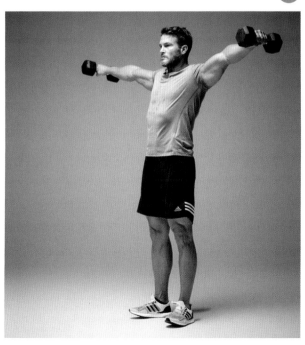

TIME 60sec **FORM** p130

6 Plank

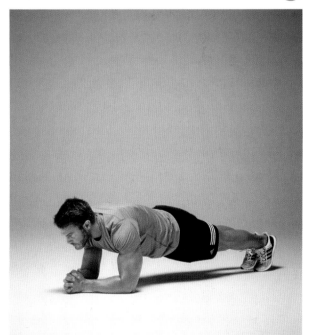

TIME 60sec **REST** 3min **FORM** p156

Workout **16**

Focusing on how your muscles move makes them work harder

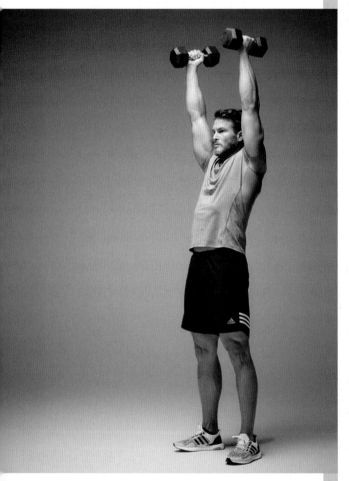

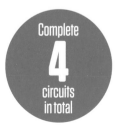

Complete

4

circuits
in total

1 Dumbbell squat

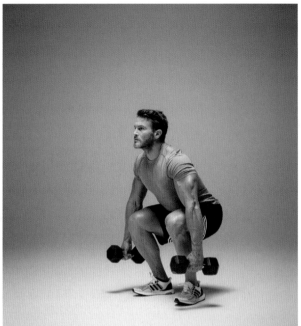

TIME 60sec   **FORM** p141

2 Dumbbell hammer press

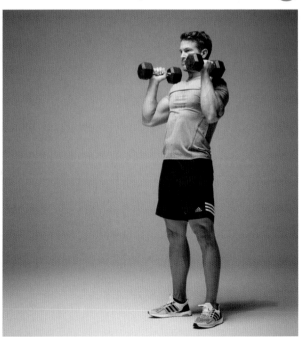

TIME 60sec   **FORM** p129

3 Dumbbell lunge

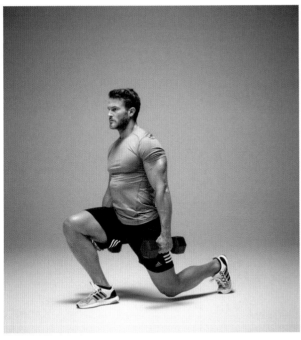

TIME 60sec   **FORM** p131

4 Dumbbell triceps extension

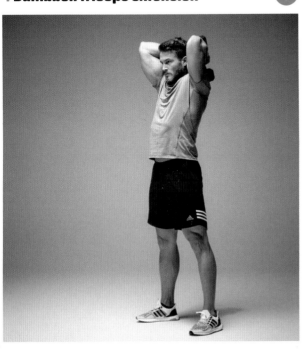

TIME 60sec   **FORM** p144

5 V-sit

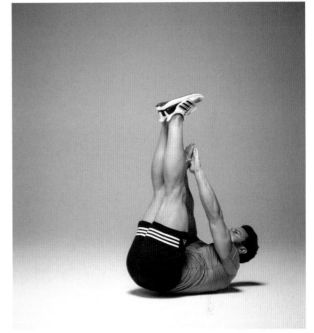

TIME 60sec   **FORM** p161

6 Side plank

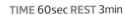

TIME 60sec **REST** 3min   **FORM** p159

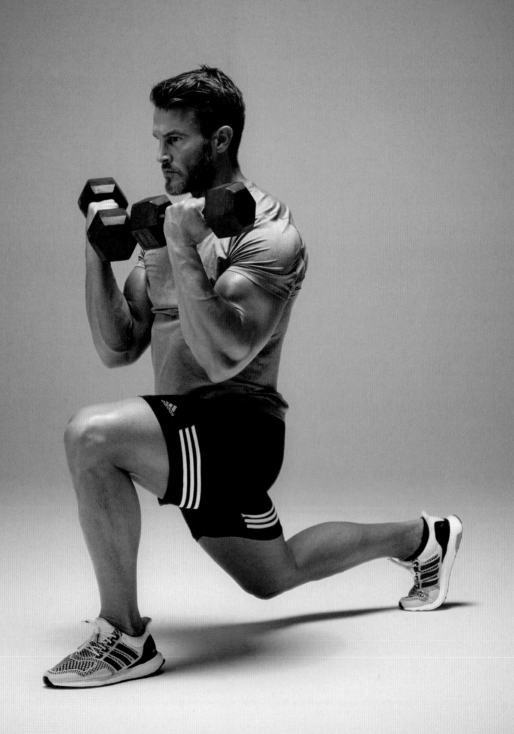

WEEK 5

You're already halfway through this fat-burning training plan, so it's time to ring the changes once more to keep the positive results coming at the fastest possible rate. In this week the four workouts are completely new, and to make it harder (and more effective) you'll do five circuits in total. Do each move for 45 seconds and rest for two minutes at the end.

Workout **17**

Do each move for 45 seconds, then move on to the next one

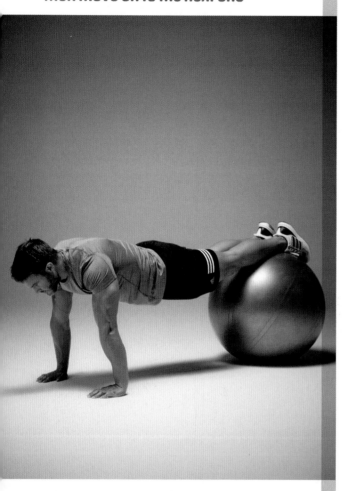

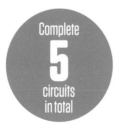
Complete **5** circuits in total

1 Dumbbell lunge curl

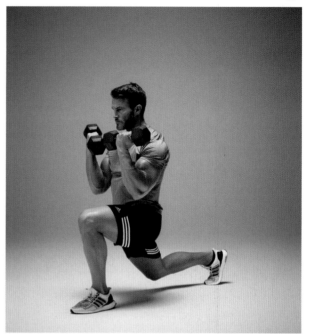

TIME 45sec   **FORM** p132

2 Gym ball incline press-up

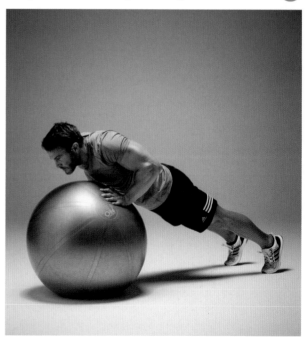

TIME 45sec   **FORM** p153

3 Dumbbell lunge

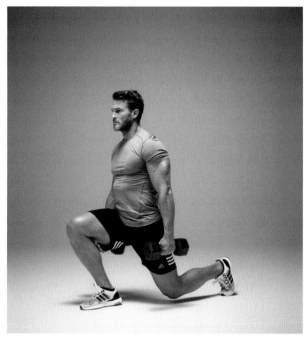

TIME 45sec　　　　　**FORM** p131

4 Gym ball decline press-up

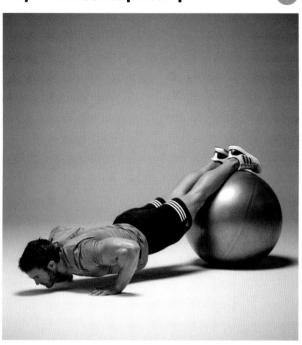

TIME 45sec　　　　　**FORM** p148

5 Gym ball crunch twist

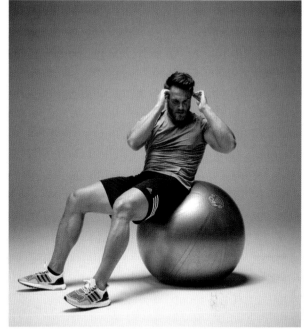

TIME 45sec　　　　　**FORM** p146

6 Gym ball crunch

TIME 45sec **REST** 2min　　　　　**FORM** p145

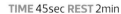

Workout **18**

Keep each rep fast but controlled to get your heart rate up

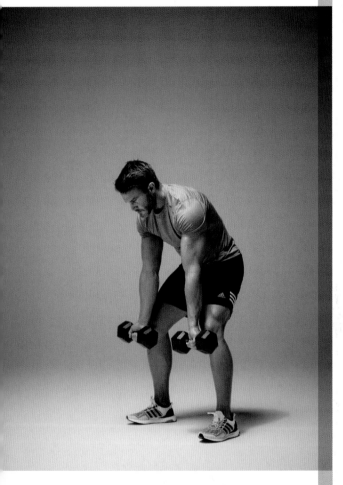

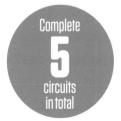

Complete
5
circuits
in total

1 Dumbbell squat curl

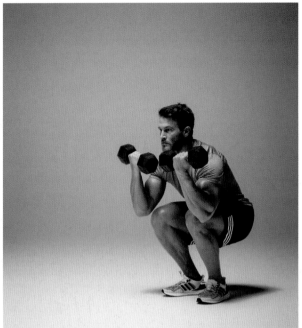

TIME 45sec   **FORM** p142

2 Dumbbell renegade row

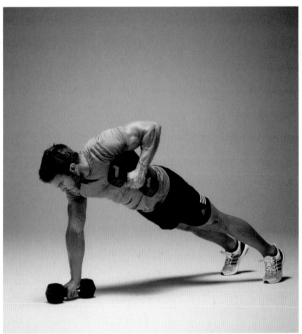

TIME 45sec   **FORM** p135

3 Dumbbell lunge press

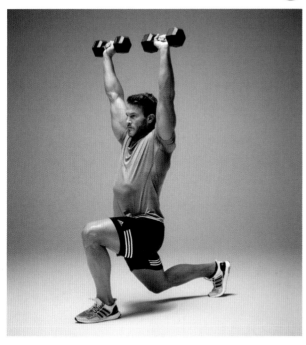

TIME 45sec   **FORM** p133

4 Dumbbell reverse-grip bent-over row

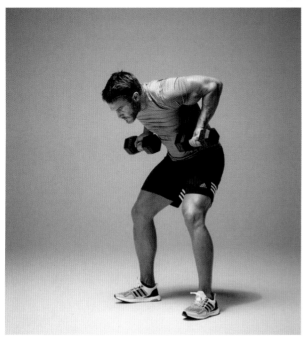

TIME 45sec   **FORM** p137

5 Reverse crunch

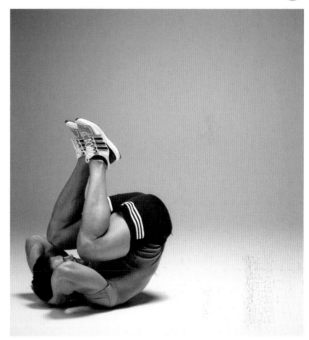

TIME 45sec   **FORM** p158

6 Gym ball incline plank

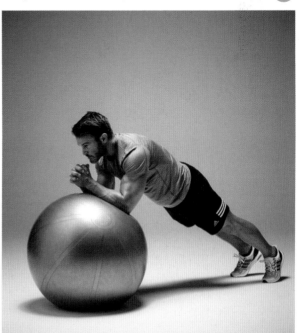

TIME 45sec **REST** 2min   **FORM** p152

Workout **19**

Try listening to music to keep
your body moving consistently

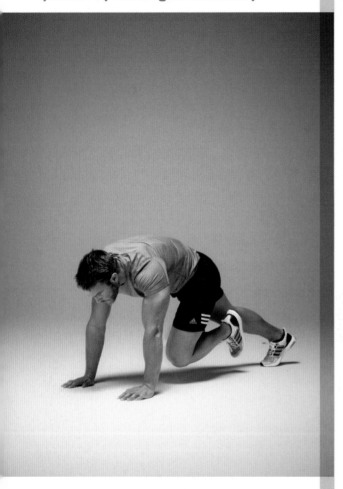

Complete
5
circuits
in total

1 Dumbbell split squat

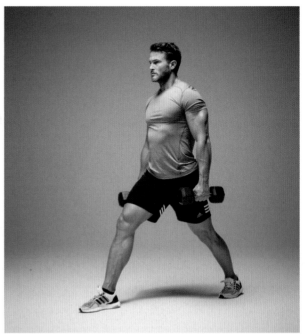

TIME 45sec FORM p140

2 Dumbbell shoulder press

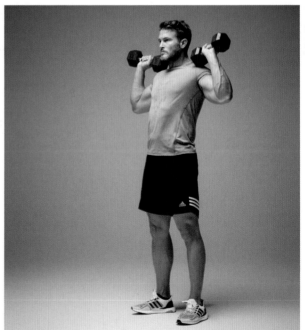

TIME 45sec FORM p138

3 Dumbbell lunge curl

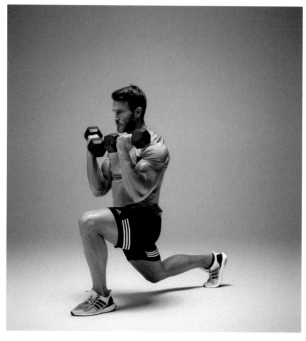

TIME 45sec　　　　　　　　**FORM** p132

4 Dumbbell reverse flye

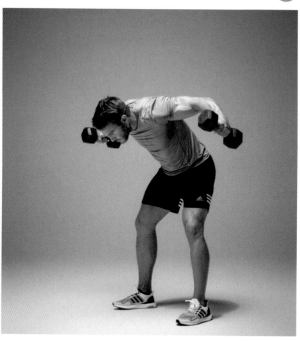

TIME 45sec　　　　　　　　**FORM** p136

5 Mountain climber

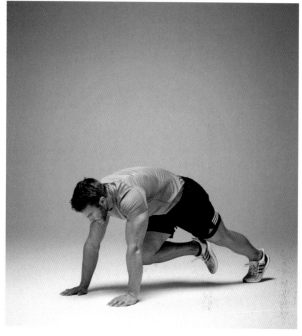

TIME 45sec　　　　　　　　**FORM** p155

6 Gym ball decline plank

TIME 45sec **REST** 2min　　　　　　　**FORM** p147

Workout **20**

Quality reps are better for your body so prioritise proper form

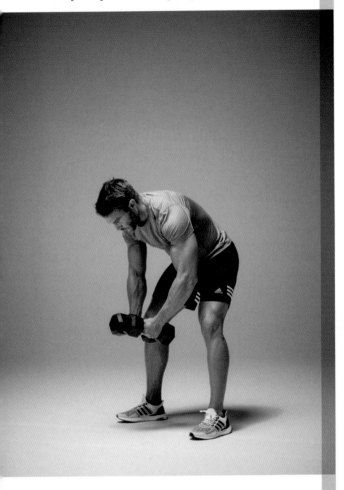

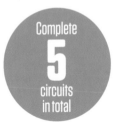

Complete
5
circuits
in total

1 Dumbbell squat curl

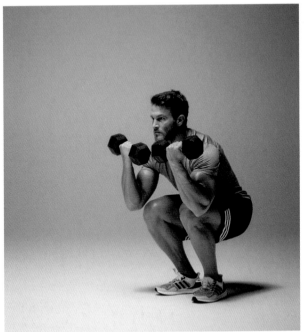

TIME 45sec   **FORM** p142

2 Dumbbell biceps curl

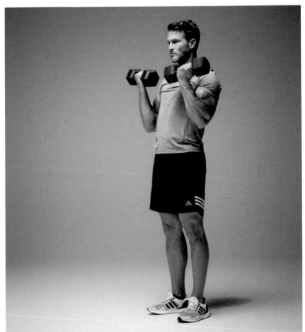

TIME 45sec   **FORM** p126

3 Dumbbell squat

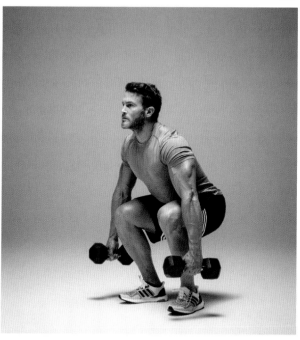

TIME 45sec   FORM p141

5 Dumbbell reverse flye

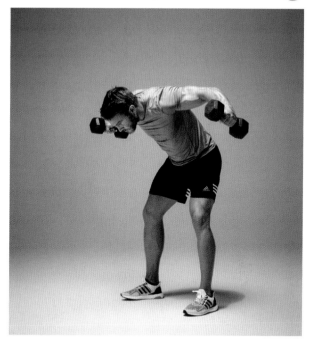

TIME 45sec   FORM p136

4 Dumbbell hammer press

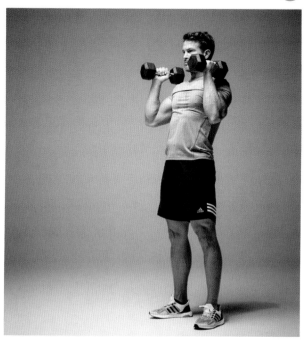

TIME 45sec   FORM p129

6 Side plank star

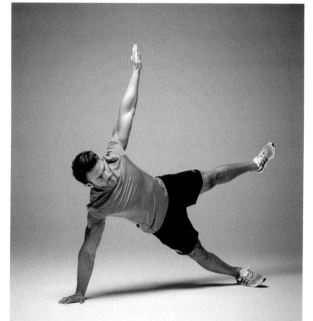

TIME 45sec REST 2min   FORM p160

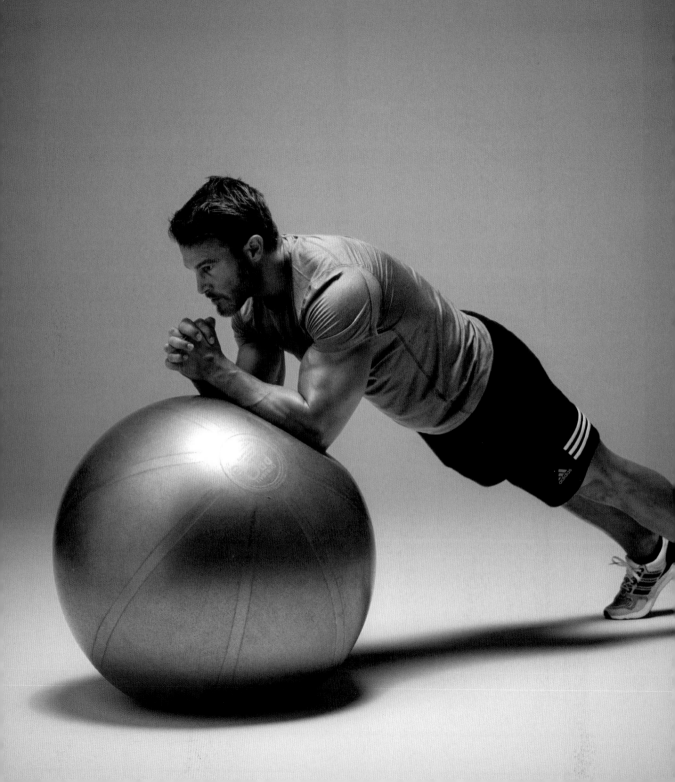

WEEK 6

To make this week a little harder than last week, which is the key to making progress quickly, you'll do each exercise for a total of 60 seconds. At the end of the circuit you'll get an extra minute of rest – so three minutes in total – to recover. You'll still do five complete circuits per workout.

Workout **21**

Do each move for 60 seconds and rest for three minutes at the end

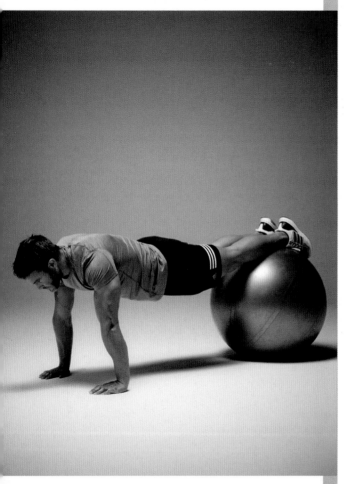

1 Dumbbell lunge curl

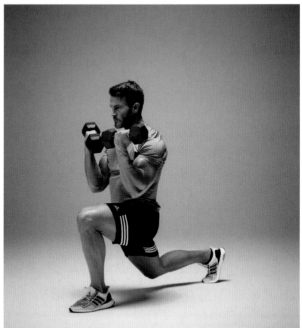

TIME 60sec   **FORM** p132

2 Gym ball incline press-up

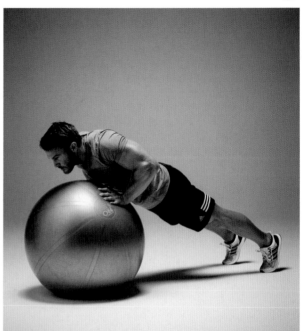

TIME 60sec   **FORM** p153

3 Dumbbell lunge

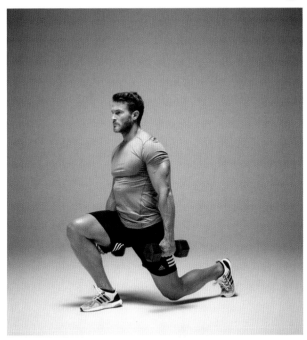

TIME 60sec **FORM** p131

4 Gym ball decline press-up

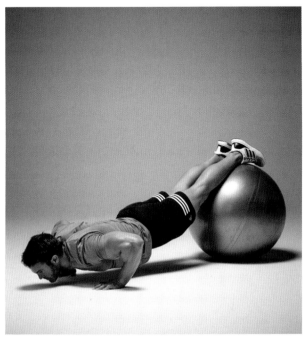

TIME 60sec **FORM** p148

5 Gym ball crunch twist

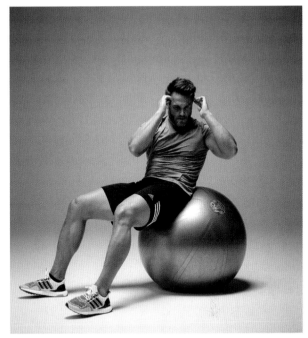

TIME 60sec **FORM** p146

6 Gym ball crunch

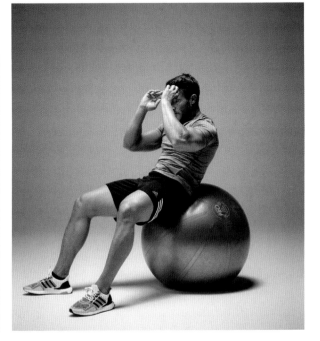

TIME 60sec **REST** 3min **FORM** p145

Workout 22

Use your rest between circuits to rehydrate with cold water

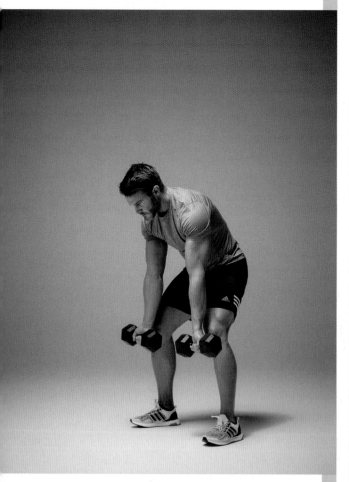

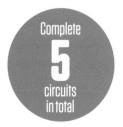

Complete

5

circuits
in total

1 Dumbbell squat curl

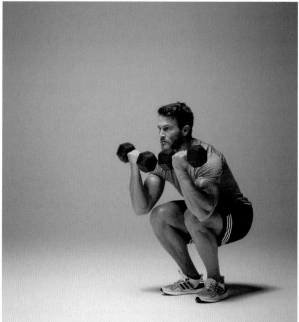

TIME 60sec   **FORM** p142

2 Dumbbell renegade row

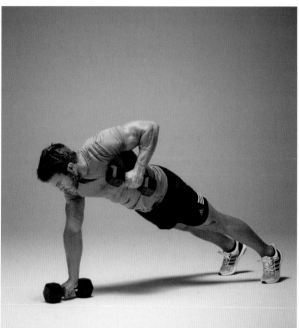

TIME 60sec   **FORM** p135

3 Dumbbell lunge press

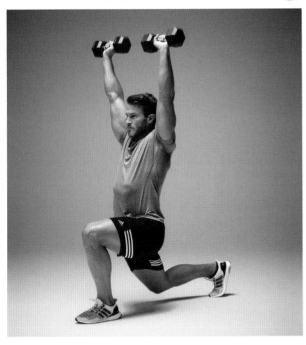

TIME 60sec   **FORM** p133

5 Reverse crunch

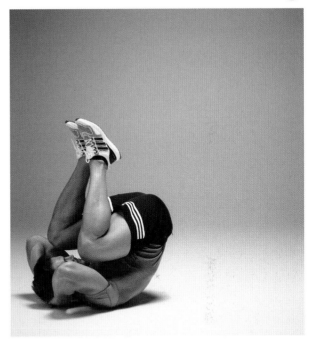

TIME 60sec   **FORM** p158

4 Dumbbell reverse-grip bent-over row

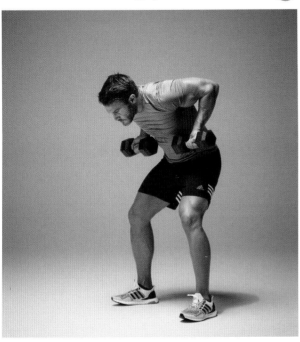

TIME 60sec   **FORM** p137

6 Gym ball incline plank

TIME 60sec   **REST** 3min   **FORM** p152

Workout **23**

Move around during your rest period to keep your muscles warm

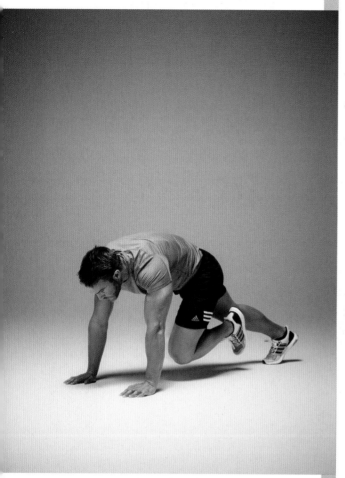

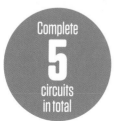

Complete
5
circuits
in total

1 Dumbbell split squat

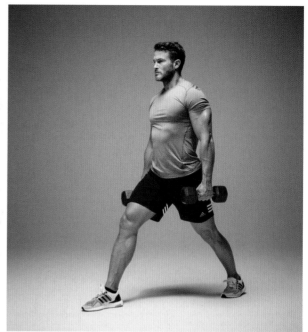

TIME 60sec   **FORM** p140

2 Dumbbell shoulder press

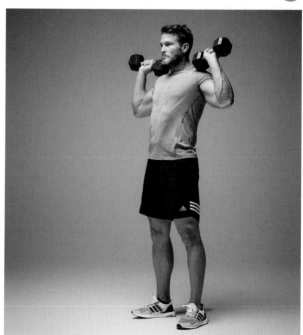

TIME 60sec   **FORM** p138

3 Dumbbell lunge curl

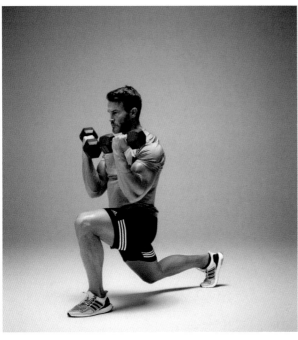

TIME 60sec   **FORM** p132

5 Mountain climber

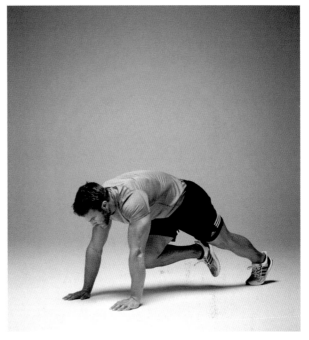

TIME 60sec   **FORM** p155

4 Dumbbell reverse flye

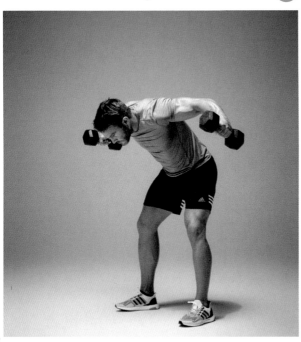

TIME 60sec   **FORM** p136

6 Gym ball decline plank

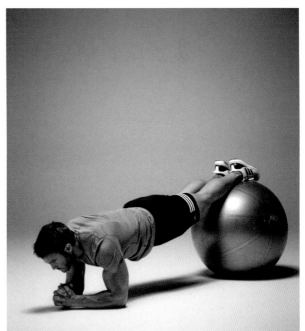

TIME 60sec **REST** 3min   **FORM** p147

Workout **24**

Remember to keep your core tight for every move to work your abs

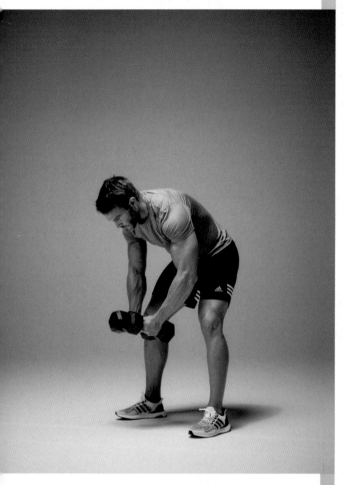

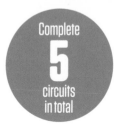

Complete
5
circuits
in total

1 Dumbbell squat curl

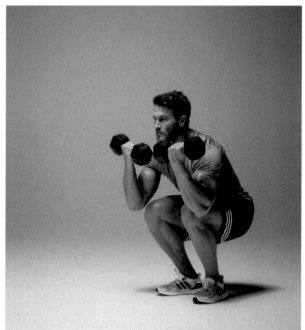

TIME 60sec   FORM p142

2 Dumbbell biceps curl

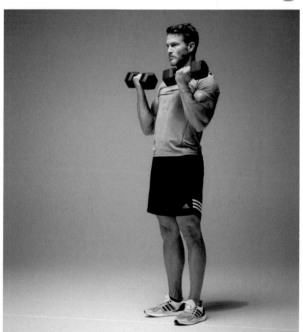

TIME 60sec   FORM p126

3 Dumbbell squat

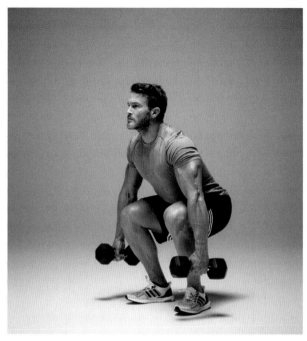

TIME 60sec   **FORM** p141

4 Dumbbell hammer press

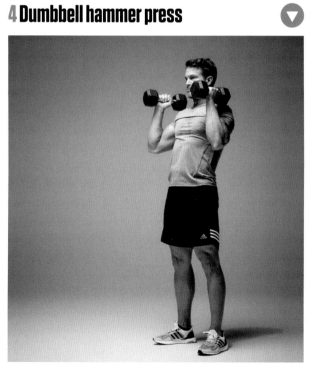

TIME 60sec   **FORM** p129

5 Dumbbell reverse flye

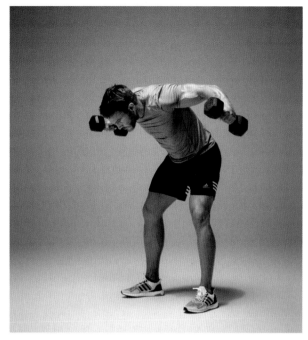

TIME 60sec   **FORM** p136

6 Side plank star

TIME 60sec **REST** 3min   **FORM** p160

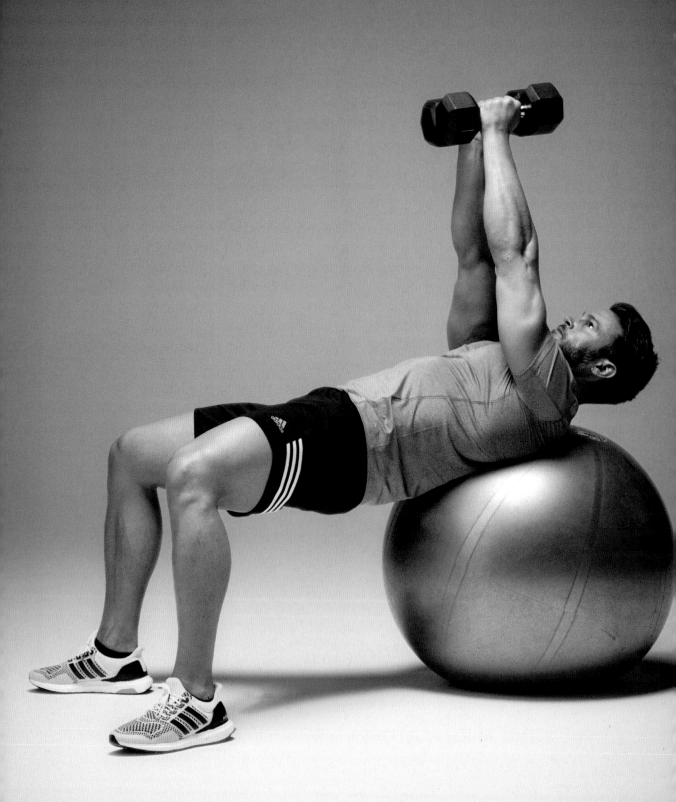

WEEK 7

It's the final fortnight of your eight-week plan, so now is the time to push on and give it everything you've got to give yourself the best chance of ending the programme with the body you've always wanted. You'll do six circuits in each session, spending 45 seconds on each exercise and resting for two minutes between circuits.

Workout 25

Do each move for 45 seconds and rest for two minutes at the end

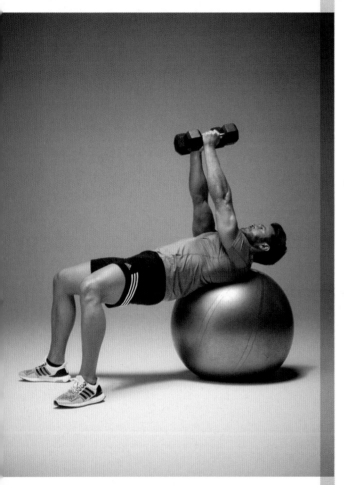

Complete

6

circuits in total

1 Dumbbell lunge press

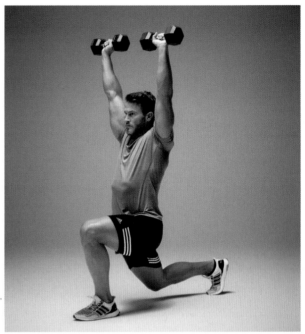

TIME 45sec   FORM p133

2 Dumbbell side lunge

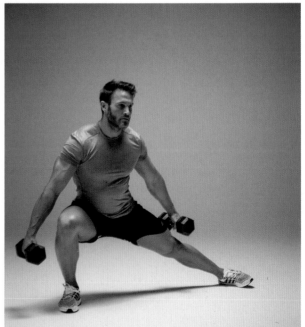

TIME 45sec   FORM p139

3 Gym ball dumbbell press

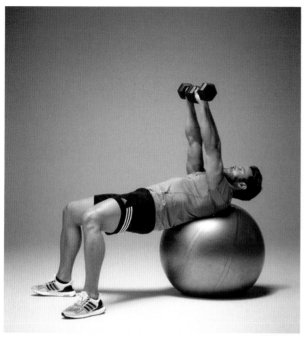

TIME 45sec   **FORM** p150

5 Mountain climber

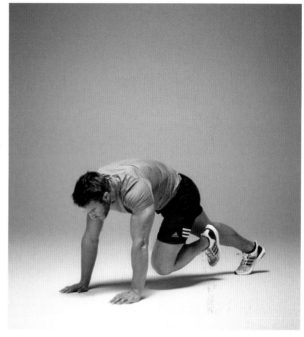

TIME 45sec   **FORM** p155

4 Gym ball dumbbell flye

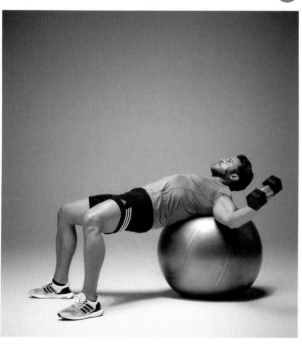

TIME 45sec   **FORM** p149

6 V-sit

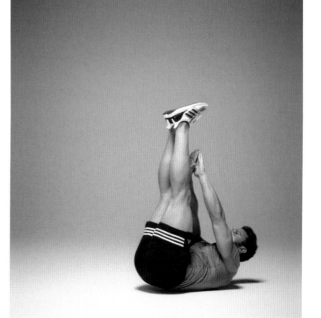

TIME 45sec **REST** 2min   **FORM** p161

Workout 26

Lift as heavy as you can while maintaining correct form

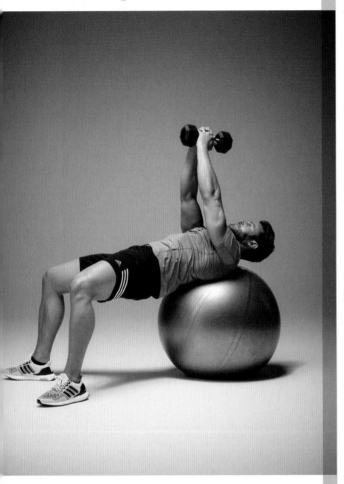

Complete

6

circuits
in total

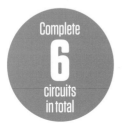

1 Dumbbell squat curl

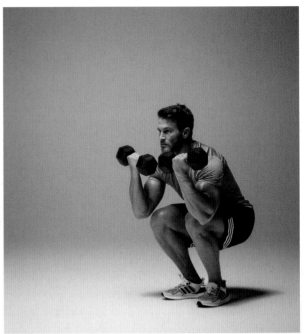

TIME 45sec   **FORM** p142

2 Dumbbell split squat

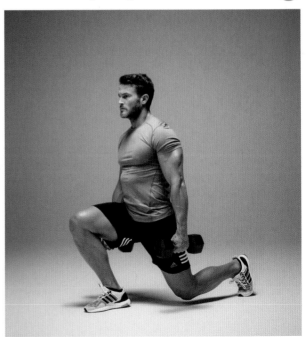

TIME 45sec   **FORM** p140

3 Dumbbell bent-over row

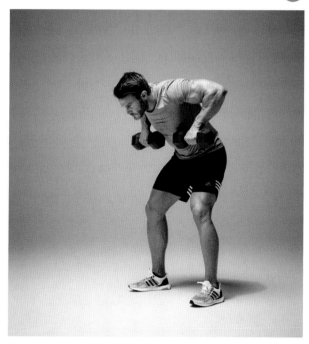

TIME 45sec **FORM** p125

4 Gym ball dumbbell pull-over

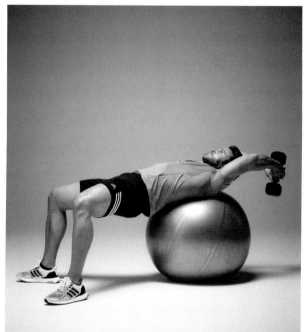

TIME 45sec **FORM** p151

5 Gym ball crunch

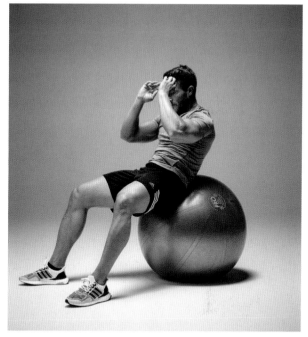

TIME 45sec **FORM** p145

6 Gym ball decline plank

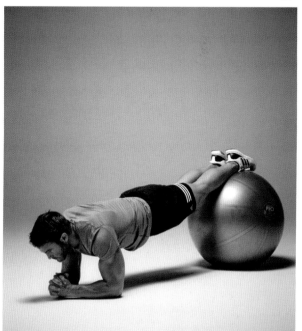

TIME 45sec **REST** 2min **FORM** p147

Workout **27**

If you're not out of breath by the end of each circuit, work harder

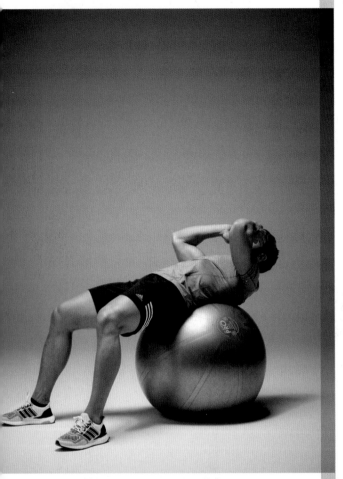

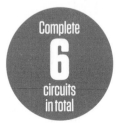

Complete

6

circuits
in total

1 Dumbbell lunge curl

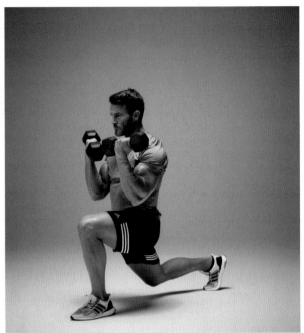

TIME 45sec **FORM** p132

2 Dumbbell squat

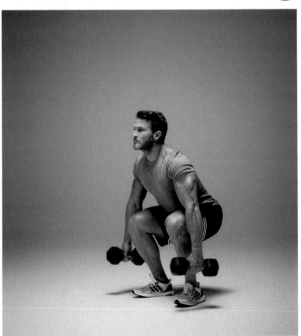

TIME 45sec **FORM** p141

3 Dumbbell Arnold press

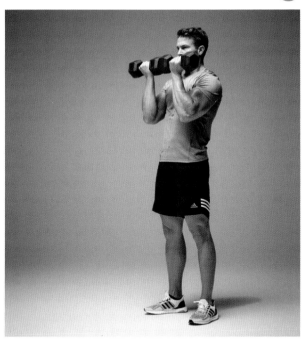

TIME 45sec   FORM p124

4 Dumbbell hammer press

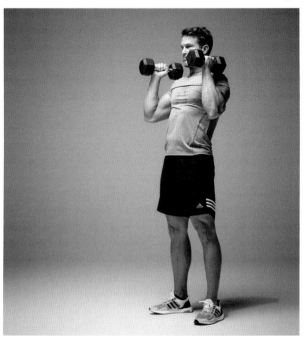

TIME 45sec   FORM p129

5 Mountain climber

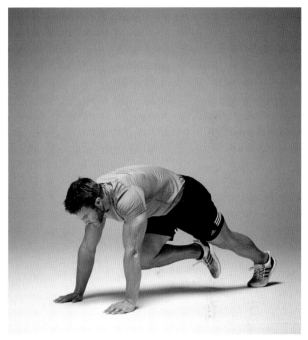

TIME 45sec   FORM p155

6 Gym ball crunch twist

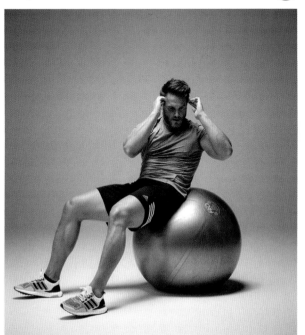

TIME 45sec REST 2min   FORM p146

Workout **28**

End the week on a high by giving these circuits all you've got

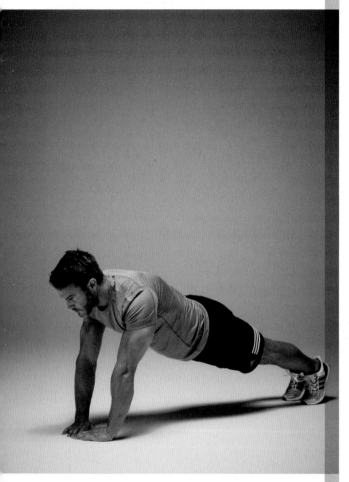

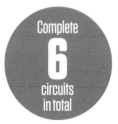

Complete
6
circuits
in total

1 **Dumbbell lunge press**

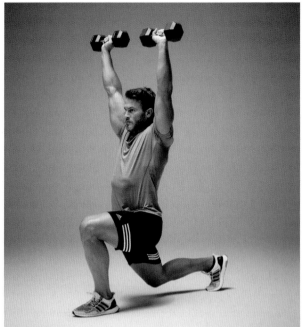

TIME 45sec   **FORM** p133

2 **Dumbbell one-leg RDL**

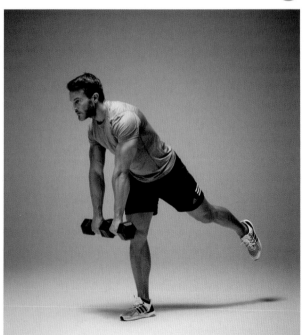

TIME 45sec   **FORM** p134

3 Dumbbell biceps curl

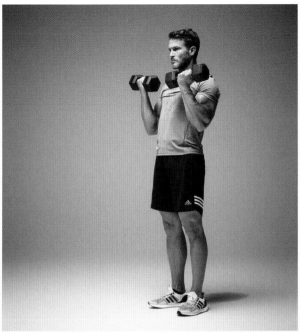

TIME 45sec   **FORM** p126

4 Dumbbell hammer press

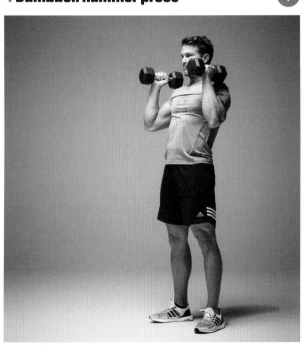

TIME 45sec   **FORM** p129

5 Dumbbell triceps extension

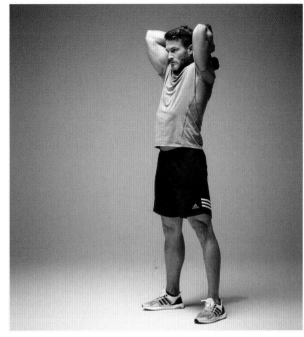

TIME 45sec   **FORM** p144

6 Diamond press-up

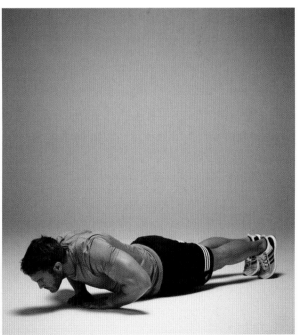

TIME 45sec **REST** 2min   **FORM** p123

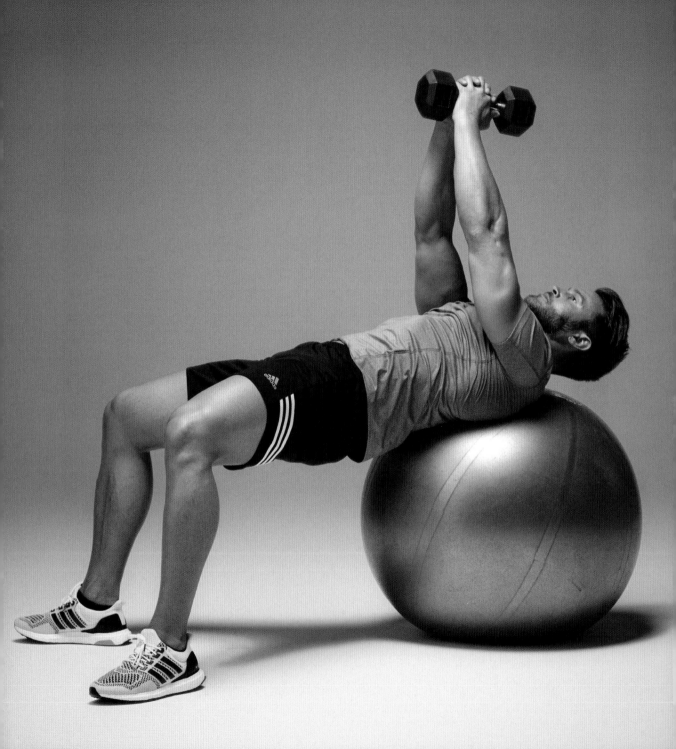

WEEK 8

The final week of the plan is the hardest yet – but to end this training programme as lean as possible, you have to keep pushing your muscles as far out of their comfort zone as you can. You'll do the same moves in the same order for six circuits, but do each exercise for a full 60 seconds with three minutes' rest after a circuit. Let's go!

Workout **29**

Do 60 seconds per move and rest for three minutes after the circuit

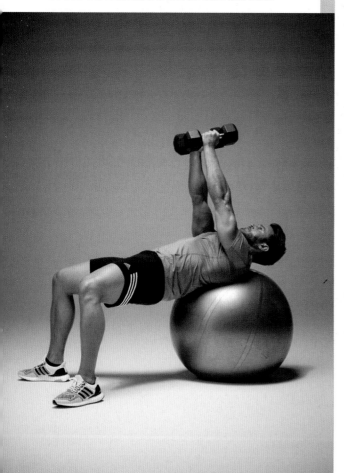

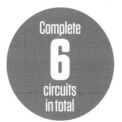

Complete

6

circuits
in total

1 Dumbbell lunge press

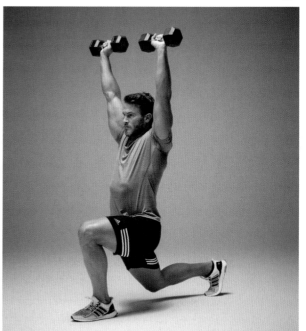

TIME 60sec　　　　　　　　　　　**FORM** p133

2 Dumbbell side lunge

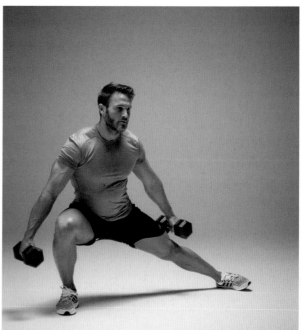

TIME 60sec　　　　　　　　　　　**FORM** p139

3 Gym ball dumbbell press

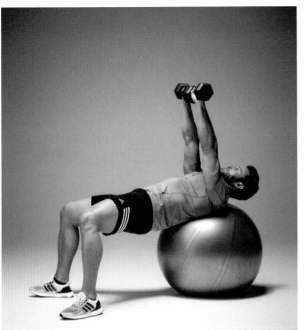

TIME 60sec **FORM** p150

4 Gym ball dumbbell flye

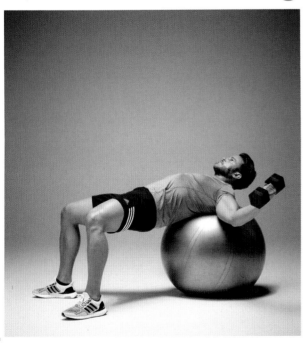

TIME 60sec **FORM** p149

5 Mountain climber

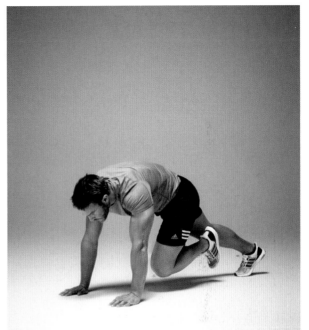

TIME 60sec **FORM** p155

6 V-sit

TIME 60sec **REST** 3min **FORM** p161

Workout **30**

Focus on moving your muscles through their full range of motion

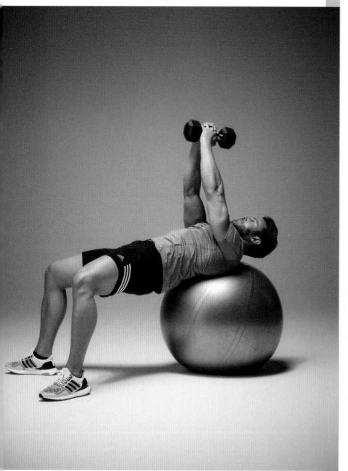

Complete

6

circuits
in total

1 Dumbbell squat curl

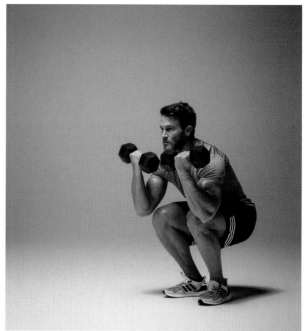

TIME 60sec

FORM p142

2 Dumbbell split squat

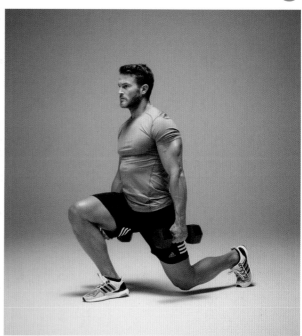

TIME 60sec

FORM p140

3 Dumbbell bent-over row

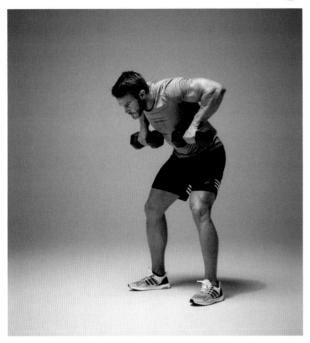

TIME 60sec   FORM p125

4 Gym ball dumbbell pull-over

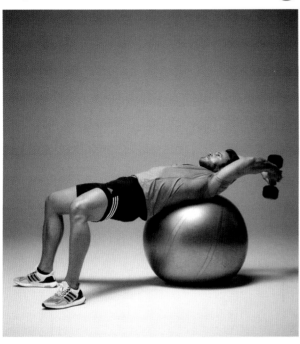

TIME 60sec   FORM p151

5 Gym ball crunch

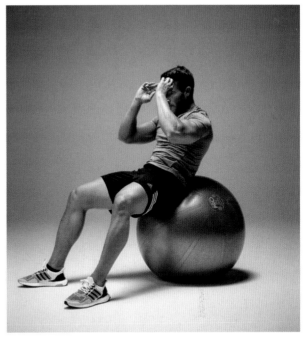

TIME 60sec   FORM p145

6 Gym ball decline plank

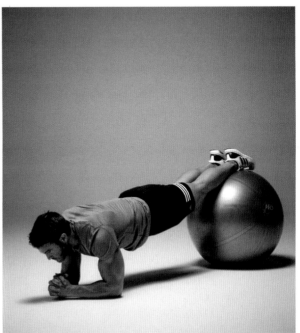

TIME 60sec   REST 3min   FORM p147

Workout **31**

Remember to stay hydrated by drinking water in your rest breaks

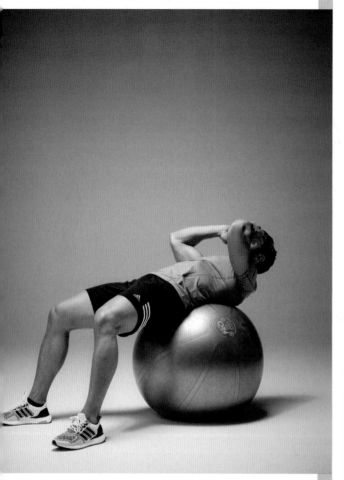

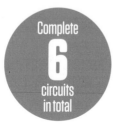

Complete
6
circuits
in total

1 **Dumbbell lunge curl**

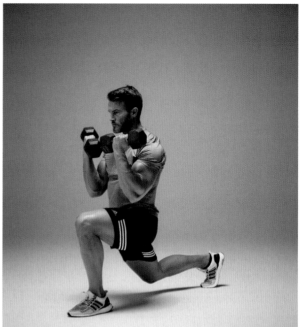

TIME 60sec   **FORM** p132

2 **Dumbbell squat**

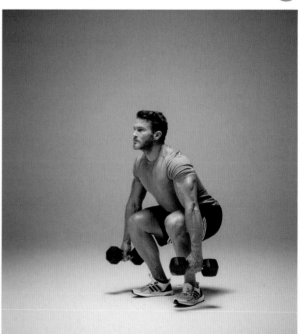

TIME 60sec   **FORM** p141

3 Dumbbell Arnold press

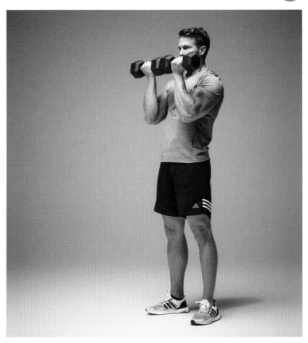

TIME 60sec   **FORM** p124

5 Mountain climber

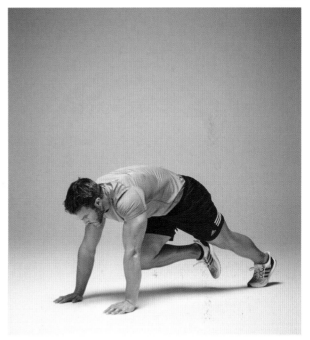

TIME 60sec   **FORM** p155

4 Dumbbell hammer press

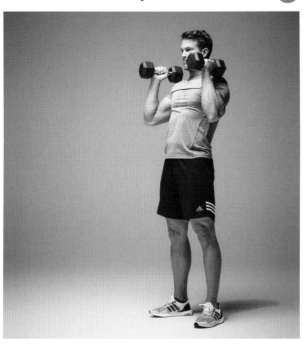

TIME 60sec   **FORM** p129

6 Gym ball crunch twist

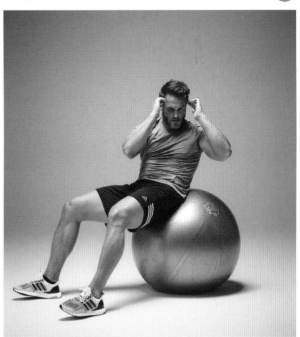

TIME 60sec   **REST** 3min   **FORM** p146

Workout **32**

It's the last workout of the plan so give it everything you've got!

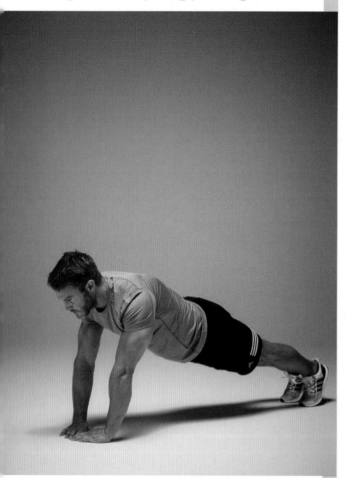

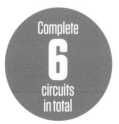

Complete

6

circuits
in total

1 Dumbbell lunge press

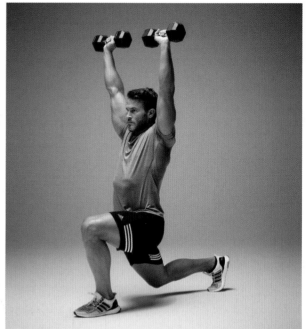

TIME 60sec   **FORM** p133

2 Dumbbell one-leg RDL

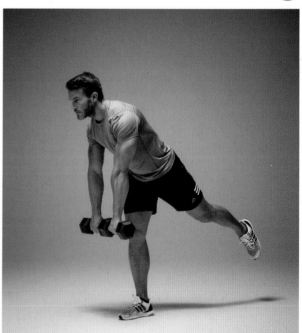

TIME 60sec   **FORM** p134

3 Dumbbell biceps curl

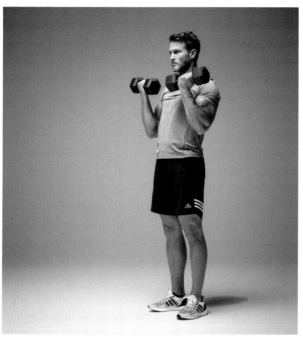

TIME 60sec   **FORM** p126

5 Dumbbell triceps extension

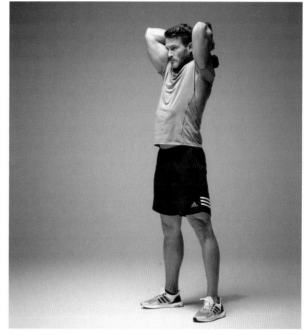

TIME 60sec   **FORM** p144

4 Dumbbell hammer press

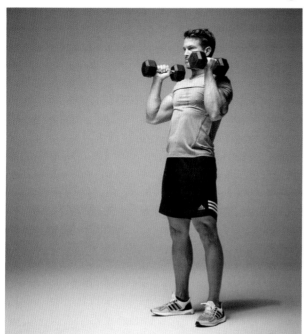

TIME 60sec   **FORM** p129

6 Diamond press-up

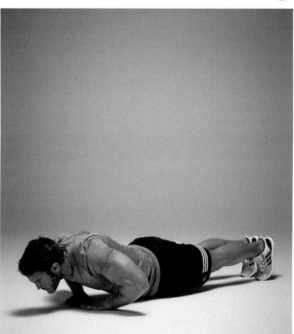

TIME 60sec **REST** 3min   **FORM** p123

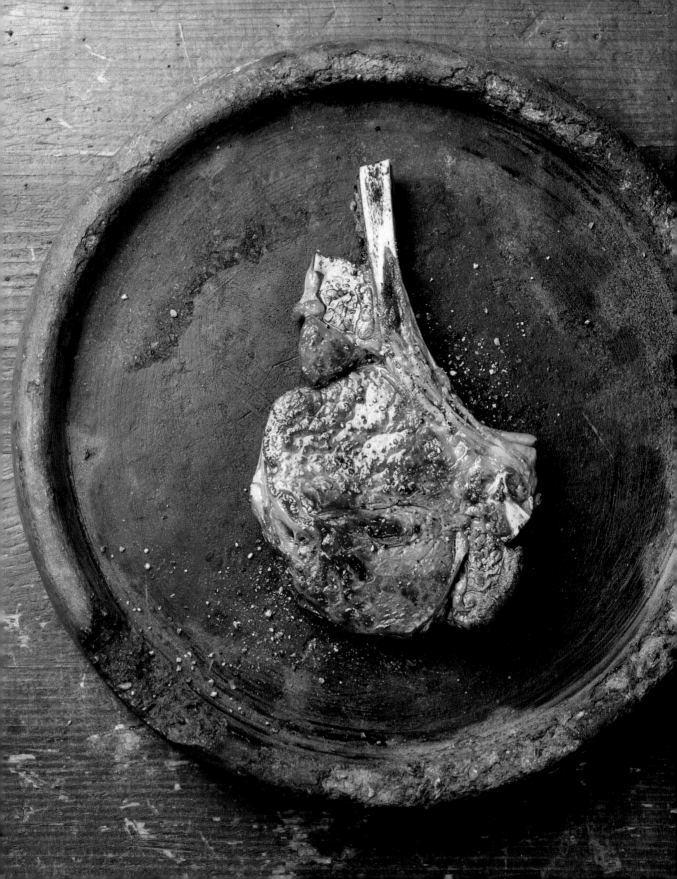

EATING FOR FAT LOSS

The only to reduce your body fat levels for good is to eat a wide variety of fresh, whole foods and follow a long-term nutritional strategy that's simple, sustainable and – most importantly – enjoyable. Here we explain how, with a few simple adjustments to the way you eat, it's easy to eat for a healthier and leaner body without giving up all the foods you love.

THE NEW RULES OF EATING TO LOSE BODY FAT FASTER

The old saying that "you can't out-train a bad diet" is a bit of a cliché, but like most clichés it's rooted in truth. The reality is that it doesn't matter how hard you train in the gym if you don't put the same time, effort and focus into what you do in the kitchen. And if you want to make big changes to how you look with your shirt off – and as quickly as possible – then you need to start thinking more about mealtimes.

The problem is that what to eat and when can seem a complicated business. But don't worry: eating for a better body really isn't as confusing as some people make out. Everything you need to know is explained in this chapter, so you'll have all the information you need to employ better eating strategies that help strip away body fat at a steady and sustainable rate.

This chapter starts with the seven nutrition principles you need to follow to start eating for a leaner body, followed by a guide to some easy, healthy daily habits you can adopt so that eating well at every meal becomes second nature. What's more, we've also suggested some delicious and nutritious meal options for breakfast, lunch and dinner, so you always know the best thing to eat – and when – to construct your best ever body.

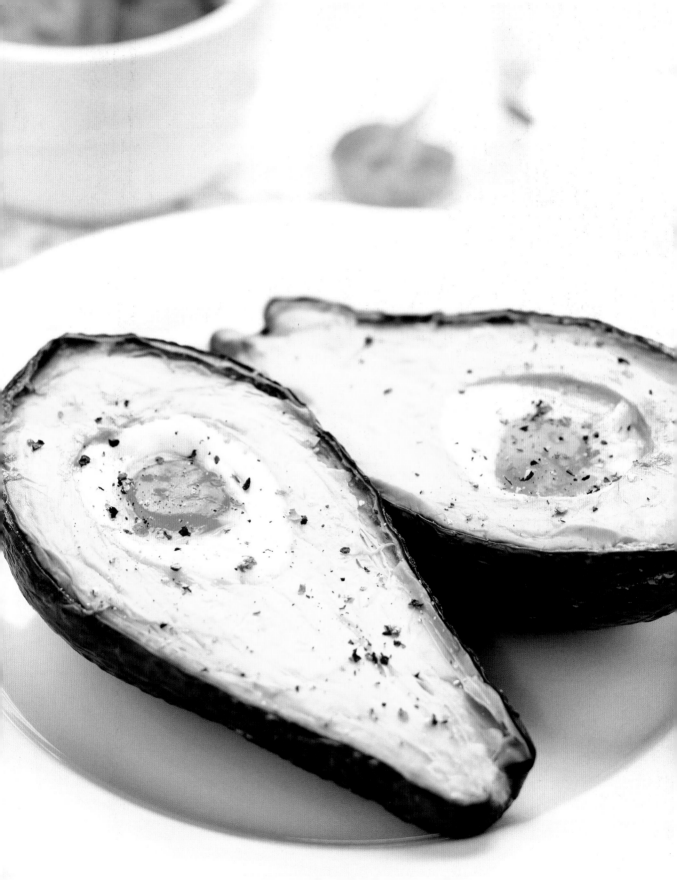

7 RULES OF EATING FOR FAT LOSS

Follow these seven fat-burning food strategies to transform your body

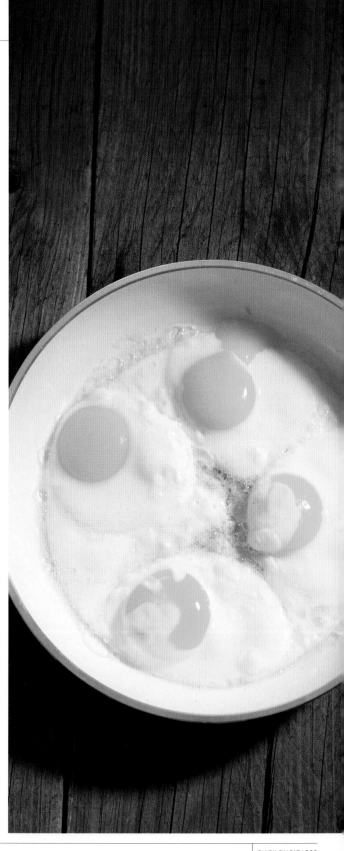

1 NEVER SKIP BREAKFAST

Breakfast, as your mum told you, really is the most important meal of the day. Your body has been deprived of energy and nutrients for the hours you've been asleep, so starting your day with smart food choices is crucial – it will help your body burn fat throughout the day and keep blood sugar levels stable, so that you resist the temptation to eat high-sugar and high-fat foods.

Eating the right foods for breakfast – and we've given you some ideal options later in the chapter (see p104) – will also improve your focus, motivation and willpower, and you need all three to ensure you stick to your both your training programme and your new healthy-eating diet plan. And if you think skipping breakfast is a shortcut to fat loss, think again: research proves people who don't eat brekkie consume more total calories over the course of the entire day than those who do.

2 KEEP IT NATURAL

All the food you put in your shopping basket from now on should be in as close to its natural form as possible. That means stocking your fridge with plenty of lean red and white meat, fish, eggs, and as many varieties and colours of veg as you can get your hands on. You'll know from experience that going to the supermarket when hungry always results in your trolley

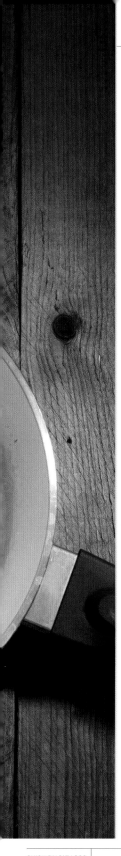

getting loaded with foods and snacks that are high in sugar and calories but low in the essential nutrients your body needs to get and stay lean.

So only ever shop when you've recently eaten, or do a big online shop once a week so you only buy the healthier foods you know you need. Eating a diet of natural whole foods, and avoiding all high-carb, high-fat ready meals and convenience foods, will ensure your body gets the maximum amount of nutrients but not the excess calories so you can start to shift those kilos.

3 THE CALORIE CONUNDRUM

For years everyone thought that to lose weight you should count calories. But once you realise that not all calories are created equal, you can't help but see the flaw in this system. Still need convincing? What's the better option if you want to burn fat: 150 calories from two boiled eggs (containing quality protein and fat) or 150 calories from a muffin (all carbs, mainly sugar)? It's not tricky – so don't get caught up in this calorie-counting confusion.

Your body is going to need plenty of high-quality protein and fats to support your exercise efforts and aid recovery so you can keep moving towards your goal. If you're unsure how this works in practice, just follow the next four rules and you won't go too far wrong.

4 EAT MORE PROTEIN

If you don't eat enough quality protein – from red and white meat, fish and eggs – then don't be surprised if you fail to make the progress you want as quickly as you'd like. The best and fastest way to change the shape of your body is to exercise several times a week, and to do this you need to support your efforts with a healthy and balanced diet.

When you work out you cause small, microscopic tears in your muscles, and you need to eat sufficient protein – which is made up of amino acids, which are the building blocks of muscle – to give your body the ability to repair this damage and rebuild your muscles bigger and stronger. Why do you want bigger muscles if losing fat is your goal? Because muscle is active tissue and the more muscle you have, the more calories your body will burn, even at rest. Aim for a fist-sized serving of protein at every

meal – and spend a little more money to buy organic and grass-fed produce if you can because it contains more vitamins, minerals and omega 3 fatty acids, which will also help you burn fat.

5 EAT MORE VEG

Let's get one thing straight – veg is fantastic. If you struggle to get your five-a-day then up your game, because you need to have veg – and a wide variety of it – with every meal you eat. It's packed with the vitamins and minerals your body will be crying out for after training, as well as fibre to keep you feeling fuller for longer and stabilise your blood sugar levels so you won't be tempted by sweet snacks.

If you really dislike vegetables there are some simple ways to make them more palatable. Try adding butter once you've plated up to improve flavour –it also helps vitamin absorption – or cook them with garlic, chilli or any other herbs and spices you like.

6 FAT IS YOUR FRIEND

Fat in food was vilified for decades for causing health problems ranging from obesity to heart disease. But the research behind these claims has been largely discredited and the importance of fats to a healthy diet – especially with regards to better hormone function, which will help you burn body fat – are now widely recognised. The exception is trans fats, which are unnatural, man-made fats found in fast food and processed sweets and snacks. This type of fat is not found in natural food and your body doesn't know how to deal with it, which is why eating it can cause all kinds of unpleasant health problems.

7 STOP DRINKING SUGAR

One of the easiest ways to boost your chances of shrinking your gut is to stop drinking so many calories, especially the nutrient-free calories found in fizzy drinks and processed fruit juices. These drinks have little to no nutritional value and should be avoided if you care about losing your belly – and about your overall health for that matter. Ideally, you should drink only three things: water (aim for at least two litres per day, and even more on days you work out), coffee (black is best) and tea (green tea is great, builder's tea with four sugars is bad).

BUILD HEALTHIER HABITS

Implement these new lifestyle routines to stack the odds in favour of blasting away your belly for ever

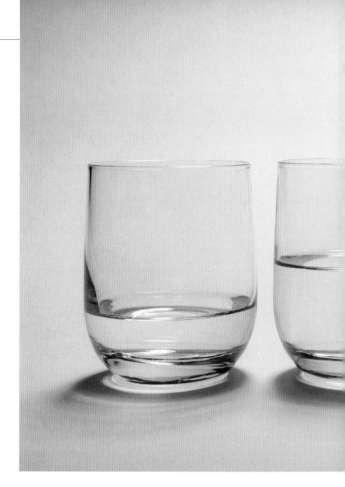

DRINK MORE WATER

As soon as you get up – even before you go to the loo – drink a pint of cold water. You awake in a dehydrated state and it's crucial to replace the fluids you've lost overnight (through sweating and breathing) as quickly as you can. Dehydration is a leading cause of poor mental and physical performance, both of which you want to avoid as much as possible to stay focused and motivated for your fat loss journey. Aim to drink at least two to three litres of water per day and more if you are exercising, especially in hot or humid weather.

Always carry a big bottle of water around with you and sip from it constantly throughout the day to keep hydrated at all times. If you start to feel a little hungry immediately drink a big glass of water; sometimes feelings of thirst are mistaken for hunger, so drinking water will keep you looking and feeling better and reduce your total calorie intake by preventing you from being tempted by sweet snacks.

KEEP MEALTIMES REGULAR

You don't need to eat like clockwork but try to eat breakfast, lunch and dinner at roughly the same times each day. To make this as easy for you as possible we have put together an easy guide to choosing nutritious meals that taste great too, starting on p104. All you need to do is choose a base for breakfast, lunch and dinner then add a variety of different sides and toppings to create the very best fat-burning and muscle-building meals. Getting into shape has never been so easy or so tasty!

A mealtime routine is important. Taking your time to eat can go a long way to maximising the nutritional impact of the wholesome food you're consuming, whereas eating in a rushed or stressed state won't. Eating at set times also removes the risk that you'll skip meals or go for long periods without eating anything, which more often than not results in cravings for high-sugar and high-fat snacks and convenience foods.

KEEP A FOOD DIARY

If you're really struggling to stay on top of your diet and consistently make the best food decisions, start keeping a food diary. This doesn't mean you need to write down every single calorie you consume, or even the number of grams of carbs, fats or protein you've eaten. A simple note of what you ate and how much of it, as well as a few brief notes on how you feel – especially your energy and motivation levels – will give you a good steer on where you are going right or what you might be doing wrong.

Much like keeping a workout diary for your gym sessions, a diet diary will make you far better informed about the foods and meals you eat, which then allows you to make small and sensible changes to your nutritional approach and keep moving closer to finding the best dietary strategy for you. After all, there is no one-size-fits-all approach for eating for fat loss: what works for someone you know won't necessary work for you, so it's important to be flexible and open-

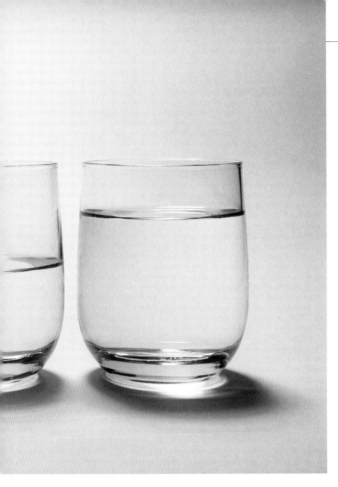

That said, you do need to be smart when selecting the carbs you eat. It's best to avoid all types of sugar, and limit consumption of fast-release carbs, like processed white bread, pasta and rice, which have been stripped of many of their nutrients and much of their fibre content. This means the energy from these carbs enters your bloodstream faster and causes a blood sugar spike.

To lose fat quicker you want blood sugar levels that are as stable as possible. So your carbs should come from slow-release sources, like sweet potatoes and brown rice, as well as plenty of fibre-rich, nutrient-dense veg. Basically, you can't eat too many vegetables when following this plan. The more the better.

EATING OUT MADE EASY

It's almost inevitable that over the next eight weeks you'll get an invitation to dinner that you don't want to turn down. But this needn't be a cause of stress or fear that you'll be jeopardising your fat loss efforts. Most restaurants will serve you whatever you want, so long as it's on the menu somewhere (and you ask nicely). So never be afraid to ask to swap a side of fries for a mixed salad, a creamy sauce for a spicy one, or even for an extra big serving of grilled veg to go with your steak or fish. Ordering the healthiest option possible will keep your progress moving in the right direction without you feeling any concern or guilt about undoing your hard work in the gym. So relax and enjoy your meal even more because you don't have to cook it – or clear up afterwards.

WIN THE BOOZE BATTLE

The chances are you will also be invited out by a mate for drinks at some point – a birthday, a promotion, Friday – but it's vital to ensure all your previous hard work isn't wasted by a night on the town. If you want to make the fastest progress possible then it's best not to drink alcohol at all, at least not until you're getting close to having the body you want.

However, if the occasion or situation warrants you raising a glass, then stick to a clear spirit and a low-calorie mixer – vodka and soda or gin and tonic are your best bet, and always ask for a big wedge of lime, because it will slightly blunt the sugar spike from the booze. A small glass of red wine is also OK, but pints of lager or cider and sugary cocktails are best avoided. For most people it's almost impossible to have just a single pint and stop, and the more you drink, the more empty calories you pour down your neck that will ultimately end up on your belly.

More than that, you're more likely to make poor food choices under the influence as your blood sugar levels crash and hunger strikes. And are you really going to make the gym tomorrow with a raging hangover? Have one drink, if you must, then switch to water or go home to avoid further temptation. Your body will thank you in the morning.

minded and to keep experimenting until you find a food strategy you know you can follow indefinitely.

TRY BATCH COOKING

When making your evening meal, double up on the ingredients and make two portions so that you will have a delicious and healthy home-cooked meal ready for tomorrow's lunch. This will not only save you time and money, it will also make it much easier for you to eat healthily and keep you on the path to significant fat loss.

An even better strategy, if you can find the time, is to batch-cook two or three different meals at the weekend and keep them in the fridge or freezer. Simply reheat them throughout the week to make eating for fat loss quicker and easier than ever.

BE CLEVER WITH CARBS

We're certainly not going to tell you to eliminate all carbohydrates from your diet for the rest of your life. That would be mean – carbs are delicious, after all – and it isn't even necessary. Remember, a fat loss diet is only effective if you stick to it, and limiting yourself to chicken and broccoli forever will see the wheels come off within 48 hours, at best.

BREAKFAST

What you eat first thing has a big impact on how your body burns energy for the rest of the day. A carb-heavy breakfast like cereal, toast or bagels primes your body to prioritise burning carbs, whereas a protein and fat-based breakfast not only supplies a steadier release of energy – so you don't get a sugar crash mid-morning, tempting you to reach for sweet snacks – but also helps prioritise fat for fuel, which is exactly what you need if you want to get into shape quickly. In an ideal world every breakfast would be based around three eggs, another source of lean protein and vegetables.

Make a better breakfast

To make a meal, select an egg base, add a protein option and complete the dish with two or more sides. This gives you the flexibility to eat the foods you like.

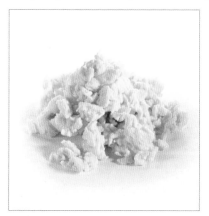

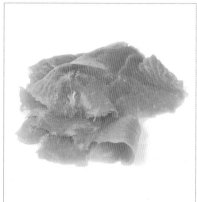

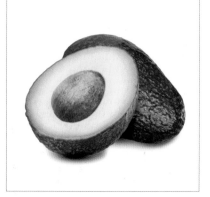

THE BASE

Three eggs either scrambled, poached, boiled or made into an omelette

THE PROTEIN

A fist-sized serving of one of the following:
- Smoked salmon
- Grilled bacon
- Steak
- Ham
- Turkey
- Grilled pork sausage
- Tofu

THE SIDES

Add a palm-sized portion of two or more of the following:
- Grilled tomato
- Avocado
- Wilted spinach
- Grilled mushrooms
- Grilled asparagus
- Grilled pepper

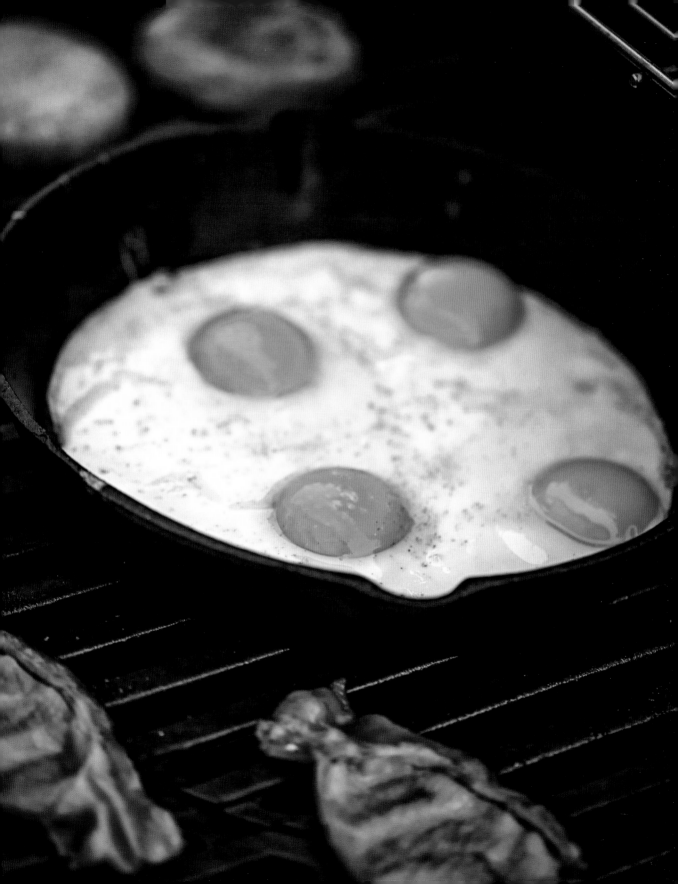

LUNCH

The perfect lunch needs to follow the same nutritional profile as breakfast, especially if you are heading to the gym after work. Your body will need more high-quality fats and protein to keep building muscle and burning fat, and your midday meal is a great time to load up on salad leaves and mixed veg for their wealth of health-boosting benefits. Because you want to maximise fat loss, avoid any form of carbs (rice, potatoes or bread). Don't despair – you'll have some for dinner! Here's how to assemble the perfect fat-burning lunch.

Make a better lunch

To make your lunch, select a salad base, add a protein option.
Finish the dish with two or more sides.

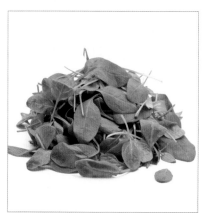

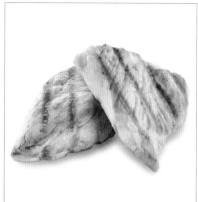

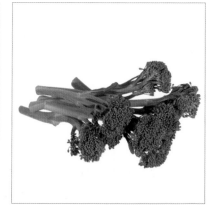

THE BASE

Mixed green salad made from lettuce, spinach, rocket and as many varieties of leafy greens as possible.

THE PROTEIN

A fist-sized serving of one of the following:
- Chicken
- Steak
- Turkey breast
- Prawns
- Salmon
- Tuna
- Ham
- Tofu

THE SIDES

Add two or more of the following:
- Sun-dried tomato
- Avocado
- Red onion
- Cucumber
- Raw pepper
- Sugar snap peas
- Hard-boiled egg
- Broccoli
- Pine nuts
- Feta cheese
- Hummus
- Mushrooms

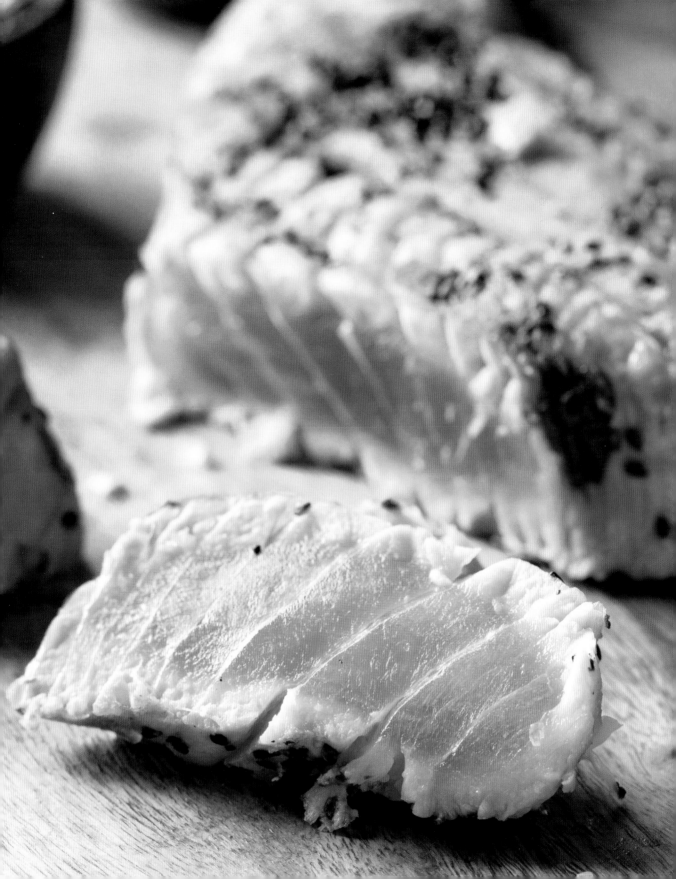

DINNER

You should always try to get your training session done before having dinner. Working out intensely will fire your central nervous system, making falling asleep when you need to much harder, so you shouldn't do it too close to bedtime. And eating a proper meal after training means all the nutrients you eat go straight to work to repair your damaged muscles. Dinner should be high in protein, with moderate amounts of high-quality fats, plenty of mixed, fresh vegetables, and a small serving of slow-release carbs, which may help you sleep better. Here's how to put a better dinner together.

Make a better dinner

Select a vegetable base, add a protein option
Finish the dish with some carbs.

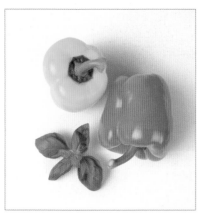

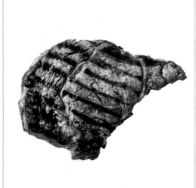

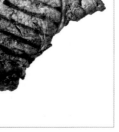

THE BASE

Mixed vegetables – at least three different kinds – either stir-fried, roasted or steamed.

THE PROTEIN

A fist-sized serving of one of the following:
- Steak
- Chicken
- Tuna steak
- Minced beef
- Turkey breast
- Prawns
- Salmon fillet
- Any white fish fillet

THE SIDES

Add a palm-sized portion of one of following:
- Sweet potato
- Brown rice
- Wholemeal pasta
- Quinoa
- Kidney beans
- Black beans
- Lentils

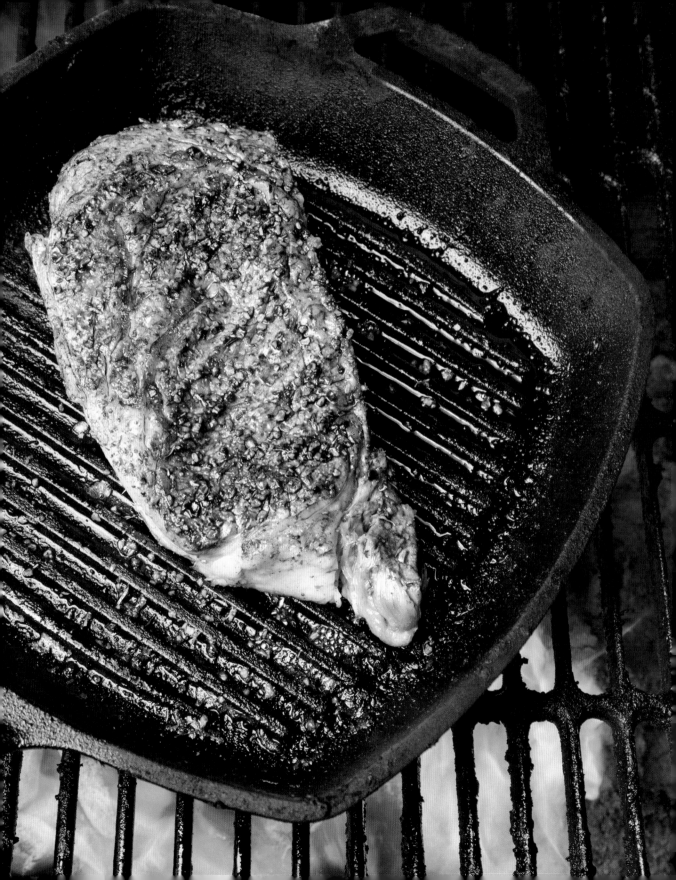

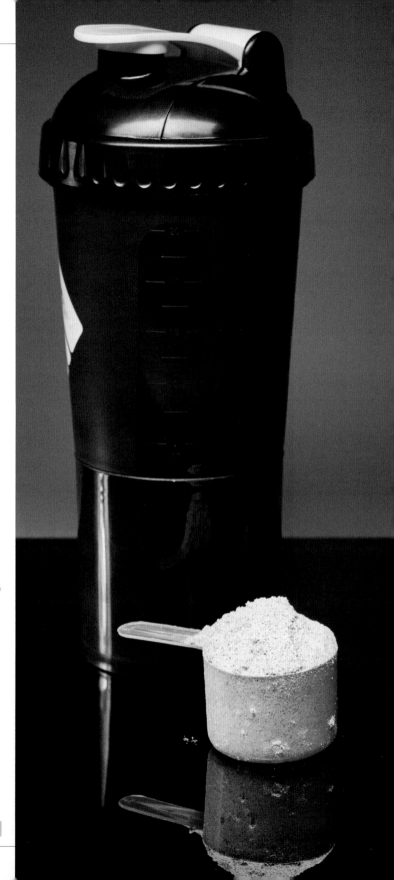

SPORTS SUPPLEMENTS

If you've ever had an isotonic drink after playing sport, drunk a protein shake after the gym or popped a multivitamin pill, then you've taken a supplement.

While there's no single magic formula for fast fat loss or an instant six-pack - if only! - supplements can play a useful role in providing your body with all the essential vitamins, minerals and other micronutrients it needs to build muscle, burn fat and function at its best. However, by definition they're designed to *supplement* your diet, not to replace food. Eating a balanced, whole-food diet needs to be your priority for the eight weeks of this programme.

So think of supplements as an insurance policy to fill in any nutritional gaps that are difficult or impossible to cover with your everyday diet. Here we answer some of the most common supplement questions.

"IT ISN'T ALWAYS EASY TO GET ALL THE ESSENTIAL NUTRIENTS YOU NEED EVERY DAY TO LOOK, FEEL AND PERFORM AT 100%"

DO I REALLY NEED SUPPLEMENTS?

Your focus should be on eating a varied and healthy diet. However, it isn't always easy to get all the essential nutrients you need every day to look, feel and perform at 100%. Intensive farming methods means produce contains less nutrients than ever before, while modern life can strip us of time and energy to prepare "proper" meals the way previous generations did, meaning we sometimes rely on processed, less healthy alternatives. Supplements can help fill in the nutritional gaps, but they should never be the starting point for trying to improve your health and fitness. For that, training, diet and sleep should all take precedence.

ARE SUPPLEMENTS SAFE?

Most UK-based manufacturers produce only safe products, but you should always do your research into a company or a product if you have any quality or efficacy concerns. That's because the supplement market, despite being worth more than £100 billion globally and covering almost 30,000 different products, is largely unregulated. Whereas clinical drugs must first be proven completely safe before being approved for general release, the opposite is true for dietary supplements – a product must be proved harmful before it has to be removed from sale.

The supplement industry is also not required to prove any of the claimed benefits associated with the product, show the safety of acute or chronic use, provide any type of quality assurance for the product, or have standardised labelling. So a bit of research is worthwhile.

HOW DO I KNOW WHICH BRANDS TO TRUST?

There are now more supplement brands than ever, all trying to capitalise on the rapidly growing market. Because of the lack of industry regulation, there will be companies out there trying to make a quick buck by peddling products that, at best, have no beneficial impact and, at worst, can be detrimental to your health and fitness.

Again, your safest bet is to do your research and look into a brand or product before making a purchase. A good starting point is to check whether the product you want to take has been approved by the Informed-Sport testing programme. Another good rule to stick to when considering whether a product is worth buying is that if it makes a claim that sounds too good to be true, the chances are that it is.

IS IT TRUE THAT SOME BRANDS DON'T MAKE THEIR OWN PRODUCTS?

Many companies, especially new ones, don't make their own products, but simply take a white-label product then add their own branded packaging. This isn't necessarily a problem if the original manufacturer has high standards, as most of those based in the UK and Ireland do. However, the longer the chain from manufacturing facility to your mouth (especially if the country of origin is outside the EU), the less certainty there is about the quality or efficacy of the component ingredients, or what undisclosed ingredients it might contain. The result can be a profound impact for athletes competing in sports where they are tested for performance-enhancing drugs (PED).

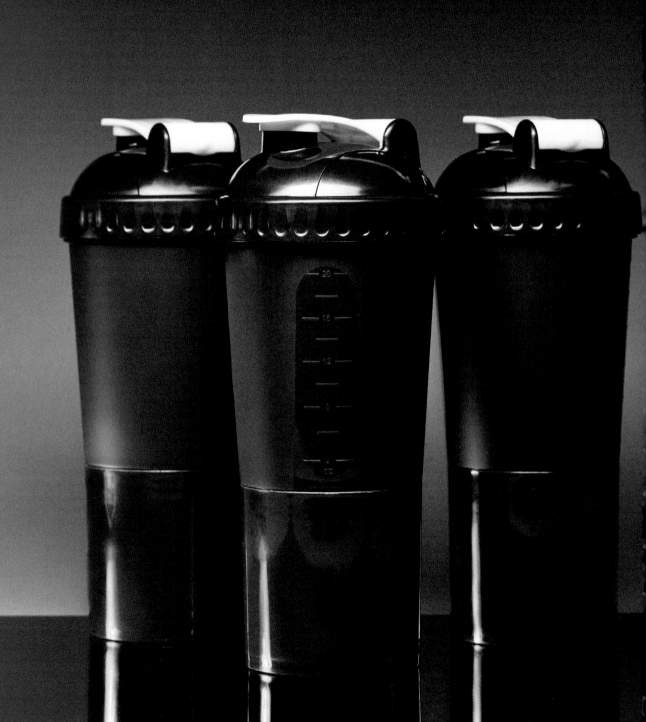

CAN SUPPS CAUSE A FAILED DRUGS TEST?

If you are an athlete competing in a sport in which you are tested for PEDs, you need to be 100% confident that the product you want to take has been thoroughly tested and approved for use. In January 2015 Welsh sprinters Gareth Warburton and Rhys Williams were suspended from competition for six and four months respectively by UK Anti-Doping (UKAD) after testing positive for banned substances following an out-of-competition test the previous June. Both athletes' defence was that they had inadvertently taken substances banned by the World Anti-Doping Agency (WADA) through the consumption of contaminated sports nutrition supplements.

Always check for an Informed-Sport logo (it contains a stick man sprinter in an orange circle) on a product's packaging. This proves it has been fully tested for all PEDs banned by WADA, and is therefore approved for use by athletes in tested sports.

ARE THERE ANY SIDE EFFECTS?

As with the consumption of any food, medicine or supplement, it is possible to experience negative side effects. Always check a product's label for substances that cause an adverse reaction, and check the manufacturer's website for a more detailed description of potential side effects. For some supplements, such as pre-workout formulas that can contain high doses of stimulants, it's always better to take a trial dose and monitor how you respond. Only then should you increase the dose to the manufacturer's recommendations.

CAN I USE THEM IF I FOLLOW A SPECIAL DIET?

If you are a vegetarian, vegan or follow any other restricted diet, you need to check each supplement individually to see whether it's suitable. The same goes if you have any allergies. Most reputable manufacturers detail the full ingredient breakdown of each of their products on their websites if you can't find all the information you need on a label. Failing that, you can always find their customer service helpline online and ask the company directly. If a manufacturer doesn't have enough detail displayed on it website, or is unwilling to satisfactorily answer your questions about exactly what is in one of their products, then you might want to simply look elsewhere.

WHY ARE SOME SUPPLEMENTS SO EXPENSIVE?

Making high-quality and effective sports nutrition products isn't cheap. But, as with high-quality food, you get what you pay for. If a particular product appears to be very cheap compared with similar products from other manufacturers, do a bit of online investigation into the company to see if you can find out why it's offering such cheap products before you part with your hard-earned cash.

SHOULD I TAKE SUPPLEMENTS EVERY DAY?

It depends on the product you're taking. Some supplements are meant to be taken daily, such as multivitamins and fish oil, because doing so is proven to improve general health and well-being. Although the likes of whey protein powder are designed for use around workouts, they can also be taken on non-training days as a quick and easy way to increase your daily protein intake. Pre-workout formulas, however, should be only taken immediately before training. If you are in any doubt about when or how often you should take a certain product, check the product's label or company website for guidance.

CAN I USE SUPPS INSTEAD OF MEALS?

Some supplements, especially in the weight loss sector, are promoted as meal-replacement products. But whether your goal is reducing body fat, building lean muscle or improving general health and fitness, fresh, whole and natural food should always be your preferred nutrition option ahead of pills, bars or shakes. These products are useful in situations where you have no alternative other than going hungry, but always remember they are called "supplements" for a good reason. Real food comes first.

KEY HEALTH SUPPLEMENTS

If you're looking for some nutritional support, these products should be top of your list

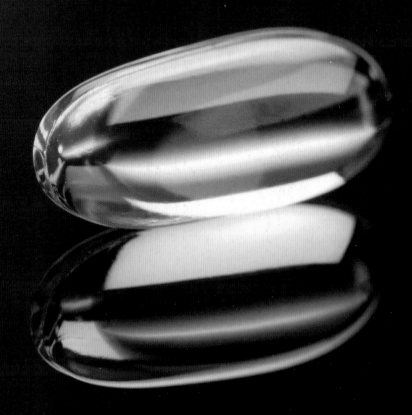

OMEGA 3

WHAT IS IT? Omega 3 is an essential fatty acid, which means that our bodies can't manufacture it from other compounds, so we need to consume it directly in our diet. It is found in high concentrations in oily fish, especially those from cold-water climates, such as salmon and mackerel. Omega 3 is crucial for healthy metabolic function, and adequate intake provides a whole host of other immediate and long-term health benefits, including fat loss, better mental function and performance, and reduced inflammation, as well as reducing the risk of cardiovascular disease, certain cancers and mental health disorders.

DO I NEED IT? The consumption of fish is an important component of a healthy and balanced diet. If you're not getting the recommended two weekly portions of fish (one oily and one non-oily) - and the chances are you're not because the UK average is only one-third of a portion a week - then you should consider supplements. And, in case you were wondering, a fish fillet in batter alongside a huge pile of thick chips and mushy peas isn't the right option to increase your intake of omega 3 if you want to burn as much excess body fat as possible.

WHEY PROTEIN POWDER

WHAT IS IT? Whey is a liquid left over from milk once it has been curdled and strained as part of the cheese-making process. Protein powder made from whey is one of the most popular sports nutrition supplements because it is rapidly digested, so it gets to your muscles quickly. When taken after training it kick-starts the process of muscle protein synthesis, where the amino acids in protein repair the damage caused by weight training, which is what leads to muscle growth.
DO I NEED IT? If you are serious about adding lean muscle fast –and remember, this can help fat loss too – you should invest in some high-quality whey powder. Drinking a protein shake, ideally made with whey powder and cold water or skimmed milk, within 60 minutes of the end of your training session will send amino acids straight to your muscle cells to be laid down as new muscle tissue.

CASEIN PROTEIN POWDER

WHAT IS IT? Casein is another dairy-derived protein but one that takes a long time to be digested by your body. This means its amino acids are released slowly and steadily into your bloodstream, supplying growth-prompting nutrients to your muscles over a sustained period of several hours, as opposed to whey protein which is rapidly absorbed. It is found in its natural form in dairy products, including cow's milk where it constitutes up to 80% of the milk's protein content.
DO I NEED IT? Its slow-release nature makes casein the perfect muscle-building supplement to take before bed because it feeds your muscles slowly to fuel your repair and recovery process while you sleep. You can also supplement with casein during the day in situations when you are very busy or travelling and face extended periods between proper meals.

CREATINE

WHAT IS IT? Creatine, an organic compound that occurs naturally in the body, is instrumental in providing energy to your cells. It is not an essential nutrient to take because your body can synthesise it from two amino acids (glycine and arginine), and it's also present in certain foods, especially red meat.
DO I NEED IT? Even if you eat a lot of red meat, creatine supplements will increase your body's natural levels to provide significant benefits. Research has shown that creatine supplementation can improve physical performance, especially for successive bursts of short, high-intensity exercise like weight training or interval training, because the energy it supplies enables your muscles to work harder for longer. Always take creatine with lots of water to avoid dehydration, and some people may benefit from taking it with food to help avoid stomach discomfort.

MULTIVITAMIN

WHAT IS IT? Exactly what is sounds like: a tablet or capsule that contains a high percentage of the recommended daily intake of the vitamins and minerals your body needs to function at its best.
DO I NEED IT? If you are eating a natural and varied whole-food diet then you should be getting all the vitamins and minerals you need. However, with the best will in the world, it's not always convenient or even possible to eat a diet consisting exclusively of natural unprocessed foods, and sometimes we all resort to the mass-produced factory foods that dominate our supermarket aisles. Besides, soil and air pollution and increasing pesticide use mean that many foods now have lower levels of nutrients than ever before. A daily multivitamin can act as a good insurance policy to ensure you regularly hit your daily target of essential nutrients.

VITAMIN D

WHAT IS IT? Vitamin D is not technically a vitamin, but a fat-soluble, pre-hormone compound that plays an essential role in a huge number of biological functions as well as reducing the risk of certain cancers, cardiovascular disease and dementia. It is produced by your body when your skin is exposed to strong and direct sunlight, but is also found in low doses in some foods, such as fish and eggs.

DO I NEED IT? If you live in the UK, or other high-latitude regions of the northern hemisphere, the chances are that you will have some level of vitamin D deficiency. One study found more than 50% of the UK adult population have sub-optimal levels of vitamin D, causing both their short- and long-term health to suffer, because the sunlight isn't strong enough outside the summer months to make production possible. (And then only if it's a good summer.) One of vitamin D's main roles is to regulate the amount of calcium and phosphate in the body, so a severe deficiency can result in bone pain and tenderness from a condition called osteomalacia, as well as contributing to many other health issues. Supplementation can keep your levels in the ideal range to help prevent these problems – but be aware that taking high doses can deplete levels of other essential nutrients, including vitamin K.

BCAAs

WHAT IS IT? Branched-chain amino acids (BCAAs) are a combined form of three of the nine essential amino acids: leucine, isoleucine and valine. They are called essential amino acids because your body can't manufacture them itself from other compounds, so they must be obtained through diet.

DO I NEED IT? Research is fairly conclusive that BCAA supplementation before, during and after training can help induce muscle protein synthesis, so your muscles grow bigger and stronger – thereby giving you more of the active tissue that encourages your body to burn fat. BCAAs also improve muscular endurance, increase energy levels and reduce recovery time. But be aware that high supplementation of BCAAs can deplete levels of other nutrients, specifically vitamin B6, so either use a BCAA product that also includes vitamin B6 or take a regular multivitamin to avoid deficiency and its related problems, which include neural damage, dermatitis, depression and, in the most extreme cases, seizures.

ZINC

WHAT IS IT? Zinc is an essential trace element for humans, animals and plants and is found in up to 300 enzymes. As such it's involved in a huge number of biological processes, including DNA metabolism, gene expression, hormone production and function (including testosterone), brain health and efficient central nervous system function. Shellfish and red meat – especially beef, lamb and liver – are among the best dietary sources of zinc.

DO I NEED IT? There's no official UK recommended daily intake, but in the US the RDA is 8mg per day for women and 11mg per day for men – but only 58% of Americans meet this target, according to the US Department of Agriculture. You should hit the target if you're eating organic red meat and fish on a regular basis, and while zinc is also found in plants, increasingly poor soil quality due to over-farming means produce is now typically less nutrient-dense than it was a generation ago. If you work out frequently, placing stress on your body, zinc supplementation is a smart move.

PRE-WORKOUT

WHAT IS IT? Designed to be taken around 30 minutes before a training session, pre-workout supplements contain a combination of compounds that claim to provide some or all of the following benefits: better focus, increased performance and improved blood flow to deliver more oxygen and nutrients to your working muscles. The key ingredients typically include caffeine, creatine and the amino acids beta-alanine and arginine, but it may also contain other compounds. It's best to check the label to be sure.

DO I NEED IT? Research supports claims that caffeine improves focus and concentration, and many people say they experience a superior muscle "pump" during training because of increased blood flow to the working muscles. For some, taking a pre-workout formula also provides a psychological boost that gets them fired up for their session and they consequently perform better. However, the jury is still out on whether some of ingredients provide the reported performance benefits, such as limiting lactic acid build-up to prevent cramping. Always test a small sample of a new product to make sure you don't have an adverse reaction.

MAGNESIUM

WHAT IS IT? The chemical element magnesium is an essential trace element. This means every single cell in your body needs magnesium ions to function, because they're involved in the production of energy, while hundreds of enzymes require its presence to work optimally. Nuts, green leafy vegetables and whole grains are the best dietary sources. **DO I NEED IT?** The UK recommended daily intake for magnesium is 300mg for men and 270mg for women. But 68% of don't hit their daily target according to the US Department of Agriculture, and that percentage is probably replicated in the UK, given our similar diets and lifestyles. Magnesium is needed for central nervous system function and muscle contractions, both of which are a big part of training, and exercise can deplete your levels. Supplementation is wise if you work out often, especially at high intensity.

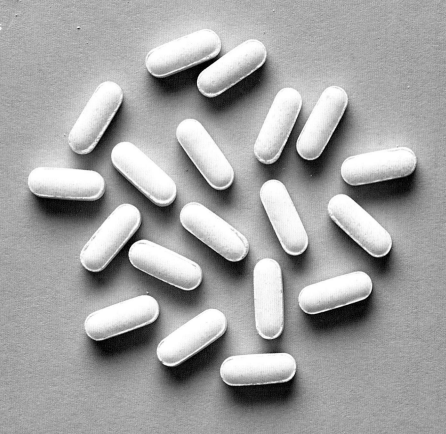

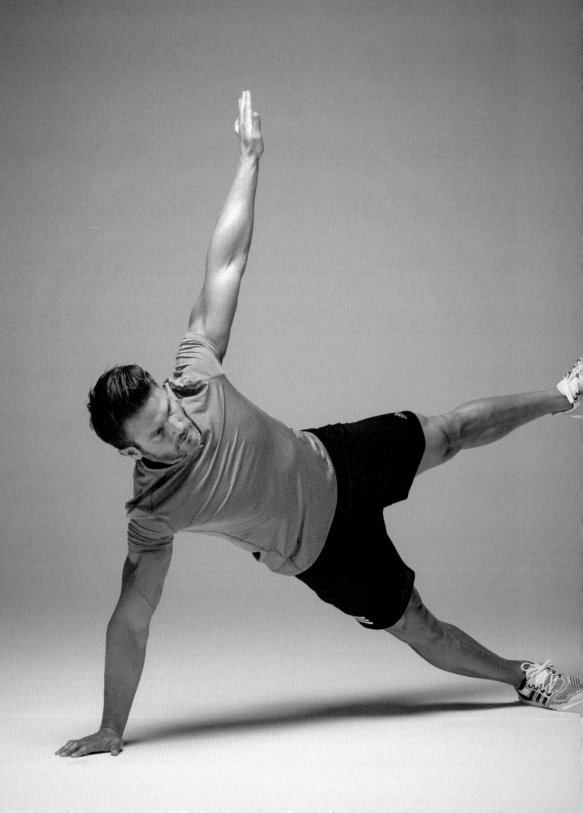

FORM GUIDES

To build a leaner body in just eight weeks it's essential you follow the exercise circuits to the letter. But more than that, you need to execute every rep of every move as perfectly as possible to work your muscles, heart and lungs harder so that your body has no choice but to become a fat-burning furnace. Turn the page to master the movement patterns of every move in the plan.

Bicycle

Target muscles Abs, obliques

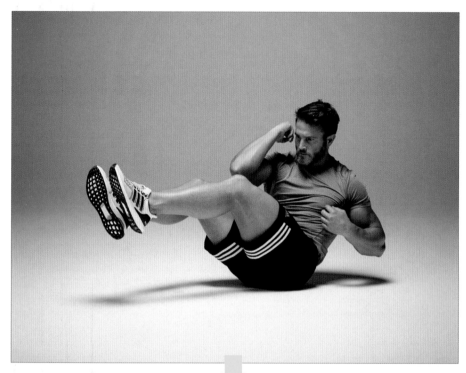

START Lie flat on the floor with your legs straight and fingers by your temples. Raise your torso off the ground by contracting your upper abs.

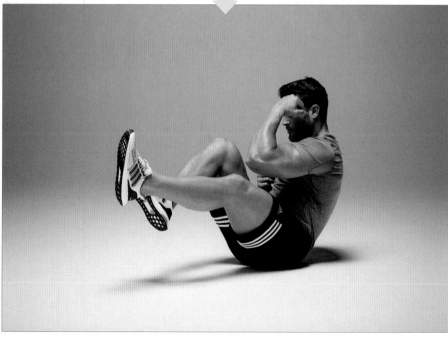

FINISH As your torso comes up, bring in one leg by bending your knee, then rotate your chest so your opposite elbow touches that knee. Reverse the movement to the start, then repeat with the other elbow and knee.

Crunch

Target muscles Abs

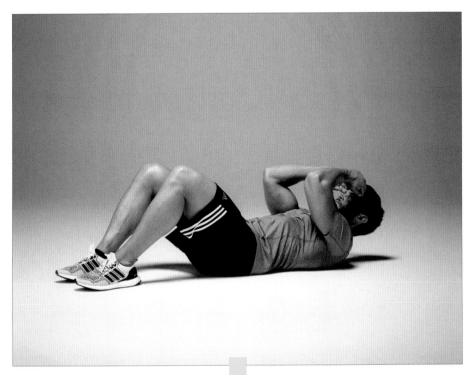

START Lie flat on the floor with knees bent and fingers by your temples. Keeping your chin up, raise your torso off the ground by contracting your abs.

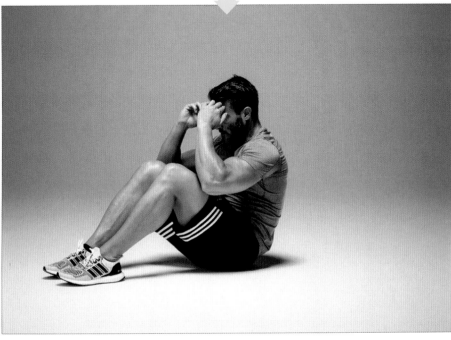

FINISH Hold the position at the top of the move, squeezing your abs, then lower your torso back to the start.

Decline press-up

Target muscles Chest, triceps, shoulders

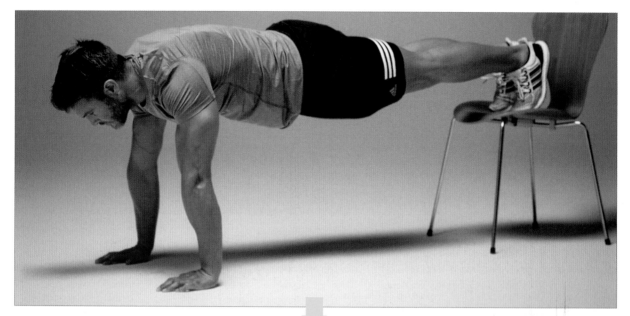

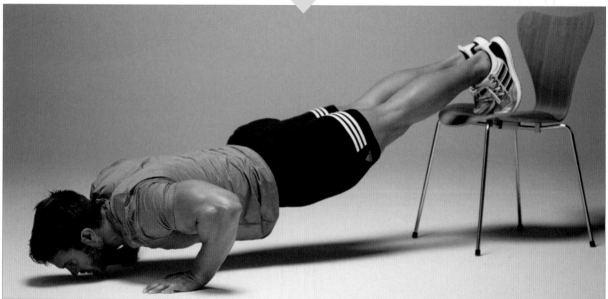

START Get into a press-up position with your hands just wider than shoulder-width apart and your feet on a box, bench or sofa. Keep your abs braced.

FINISH Lower your body until your chest touches the floor and then press back up.

Diamond press-up

Target muscles Triceps, chest, shoulders

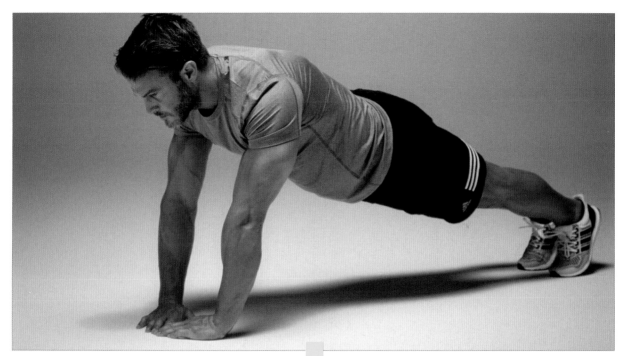

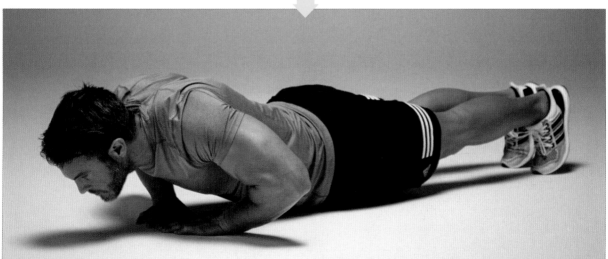

START Start in a press-up position but with your thumbs and forefingers together to form a diamond shape. Keep your core braced.

FINISH Lower your chest to the floor, keeping your elbows close to your sides, then press back up.

Dumbbell Arnold press

Target muscles **Shoulders, triceps**

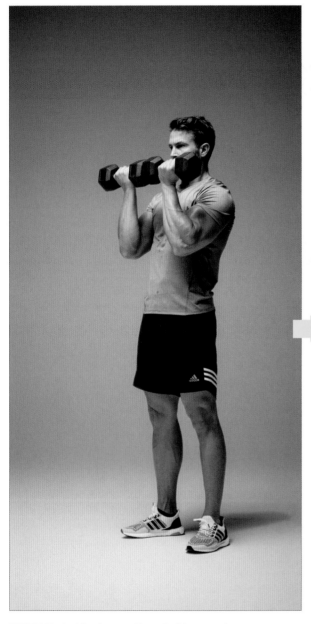

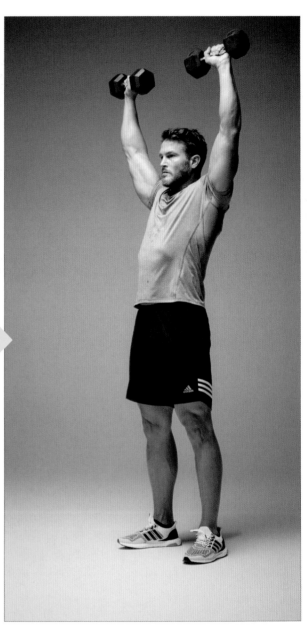

START Start at the top position of a biceps curl, holding the dumbbells with palms facing you and your elbows tight to your sides.

FINISH Allow your palms to rotate as you press the dumbbells overhead, finishing with your palms facing away from you. Reverse the movement as you lower the dumbbells back to the start.

124

Dumbbell bent-over row

Target muscles **Back, biceps**

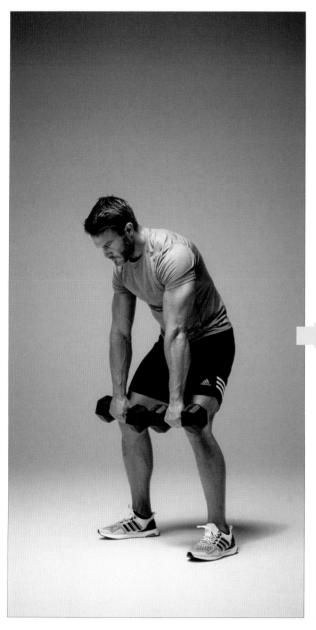

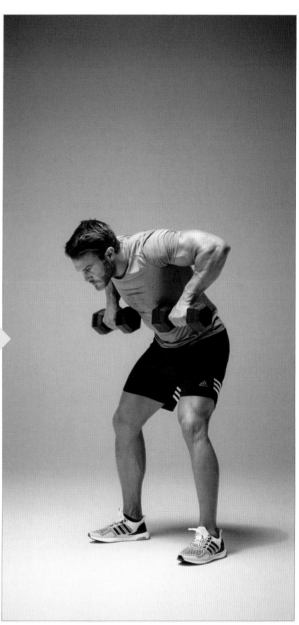

START Stand with your core braced, your back straight and your shoulder blades retracted, holding a set of dumbbells. Bend your knees slightly and lean forwards from the hips.

FINISH Row the dumbbells up, leading with your elbows, until they almost touch your chest. Pause, then lower them back to the start under control.

Dumbbell biceps curl

Target muscles Biceps

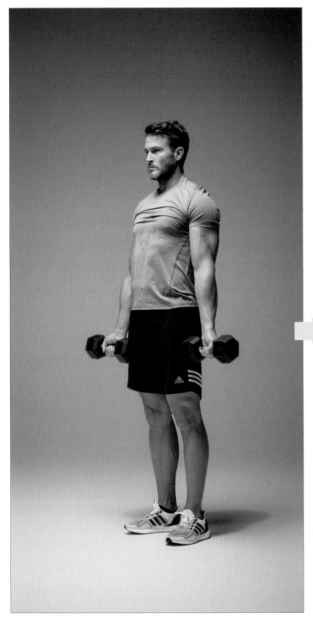 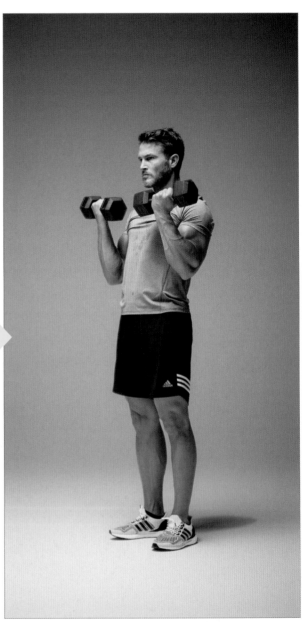

START Stand tall with your shoulders back and feet close together, holding a pair of dumbbells with hands just outside your hips and palms facing forwards.

FINISH Keeping your elbows tucked in to your sides, curl the dumbbells up towards your chest, stopping just before your forearms reach vertical. Lower under control to return to the start position.

Dumbbell crunch

Target muscles **Abs**

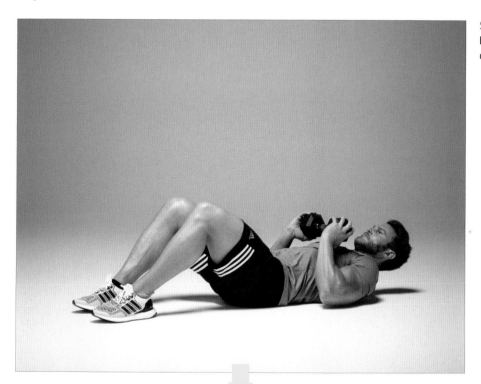

START Lie flat on your back with knees bent and a dumbbell held at chest level.

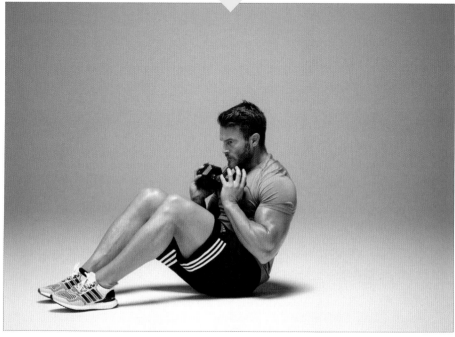

FINISH Contract your abs to lift your shoulders off the floor and curl your chest towards your knees. Pause at the top of the move and squeeze your abs, then lower slowly back to the start

Dumbbell front raise

Target muscles Shoulders

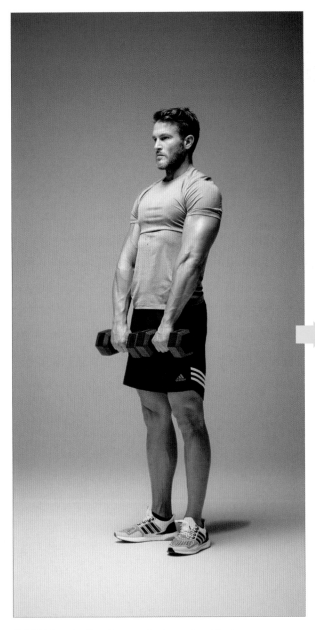

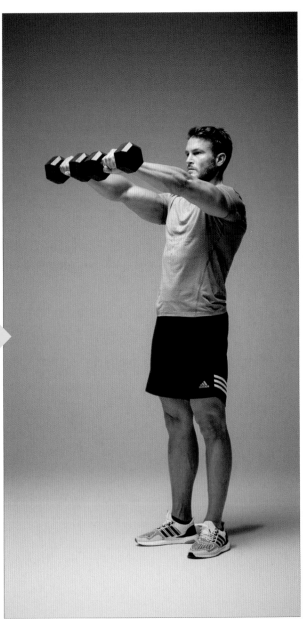

START Stand tall with your abs braced and feet apart, holding a light dumbbell in each hand by your sides with your palms facing each other.

FINISH Keeping a slight bend in your elbows, raise the weights in front of you, making sure you use your muscles and not momentum. Stop at shoulder height, pause for one second, and then slowly return to the start.

Dumbbell hammer press

Target muscles **Shoulders, triceps**

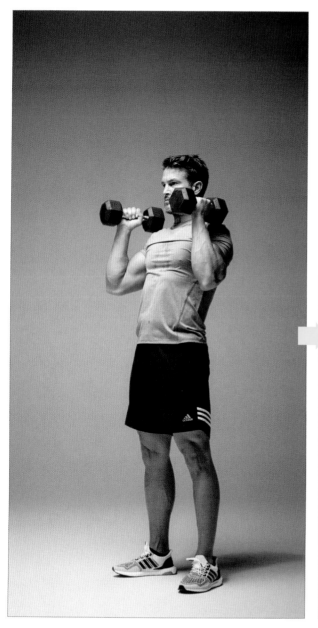

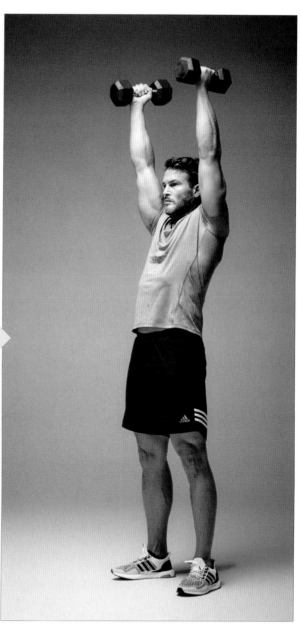

START With your feet shoulder-width apart, hold a dumbbell in each hand at shoulder height with palms facing each other. Keep your chest upright and your core muscles braced.

FINISH Press the weights directly upwards, keeping your core braced, until your arms are fully extended overhead. Lower slowly back to the start.

Dumbbell lateral raise

Target muscles Shoulders

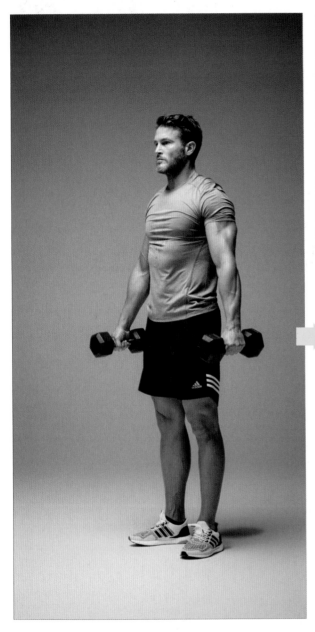

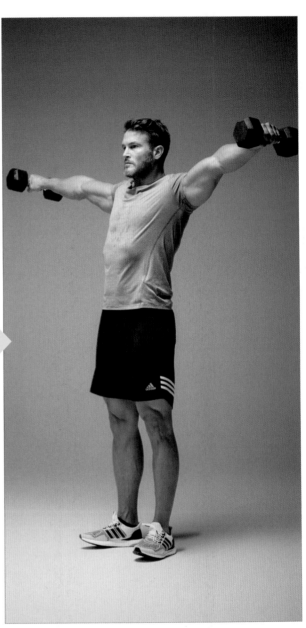

START Stand tall with your abs braced and feet close but not together, holding a light dumbbell in each hand by your sides with your palms facing each other.

FINISH Keeping a slight bend in your elbows, raise the weights out to the sides, making sure you use your muscles and not momentum. Stop just below shoulder height, then lower back to the start.

Dumbbell lunge

Target muscles Legs, core

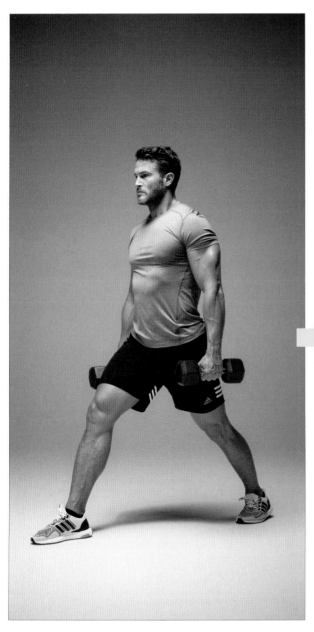

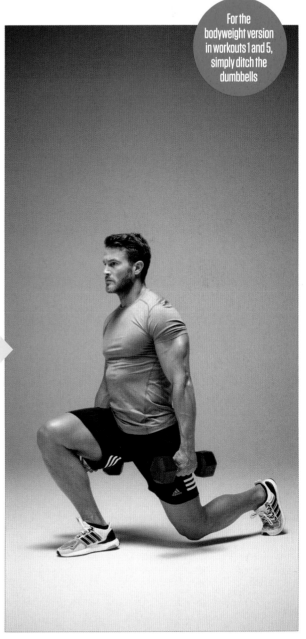

For the bodyweight version in workouts 1 and 5, simply ditch the dumbbells

START Stand tall, holding a dumbbell in each hand with your chest up and core braced.

FINISH Take a big step forwards and lower your body until both knees are bent at right angles. Push off your front foot to reverse the movement, then repeat, leading with your other leg. Continue alternating.

Dumbbell lunge curl

Target muscles **Legs, biceps, core**

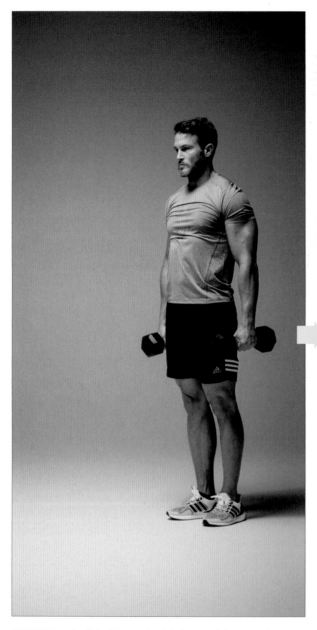 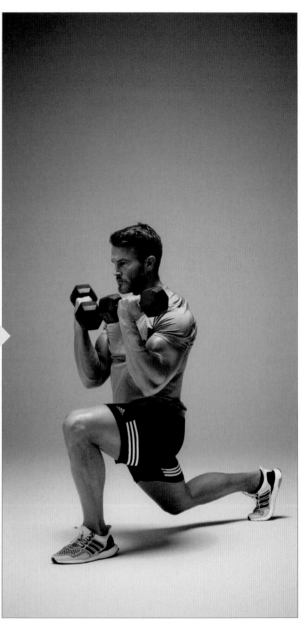

START Stand tall, holding a dumbbell in each hand with your chest up and core braced. Take a big step forwards and lower your body until both knees are bent at right angles.

FINISH As you lunge down, curl the dumbbells up to shoulder height. Push off your front foot to reverse the movement, lowering the weights as you do. Repeat, leading with your other leg. Continue alternating.

Dumbbell lunge press

Target muscles Legs, shoulders, triceps, core

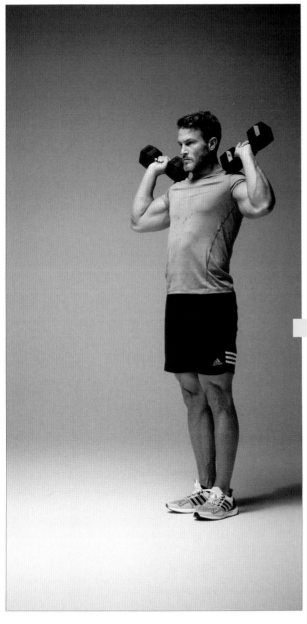

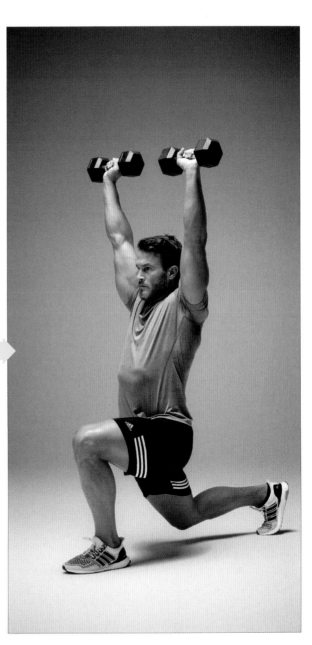

START Stand tall, holding a dumbbell in each hand with your chest up and core braced. Take a big step forwards and lower your body until both knees are bent at right angles.

FINISH As you lunge down, press the dumbbells directly overhead. Push off your front foot to reverse the movement, lowering the weights as you do. Repeat, leading with your other leg. Continue alternating.

Dumbbell one-leg Romanian deadlift

Target muscles **Legs, core**

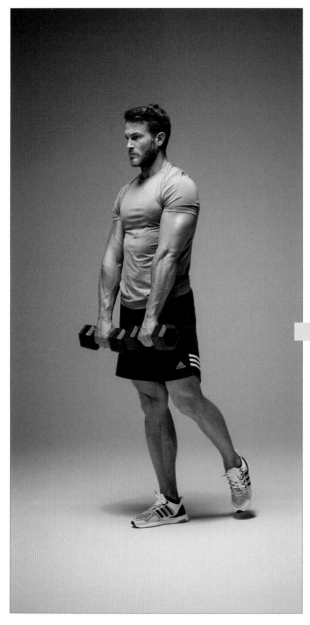 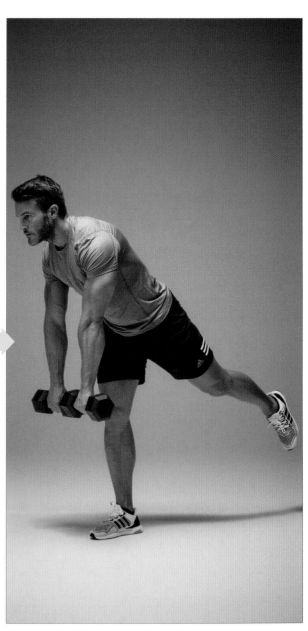

START Stand tall, holding a dumbbell in each hand with one foot off the ground. Keep your core braced and both legs straight.

FINISH Slowly bend forwards so the dumbbells travel down the front of your standing leg until you feel a good stretch in your hamstrings. Lift your raised leg behind you. Reverse the movement back to the start. After half the time has elapsed, switch legs.

Dumbbell renegade row

Target muscles **Back, biceps, core**

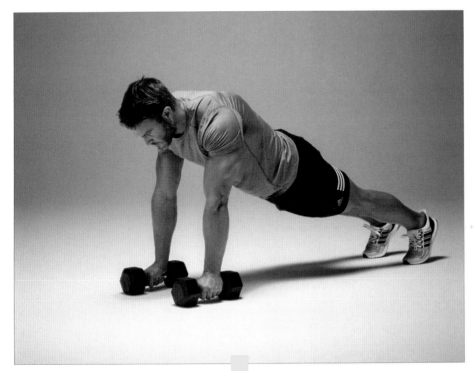

START Start in a press-up position, holding the handles of a pair of dumbbells with your core and glutes engaged.

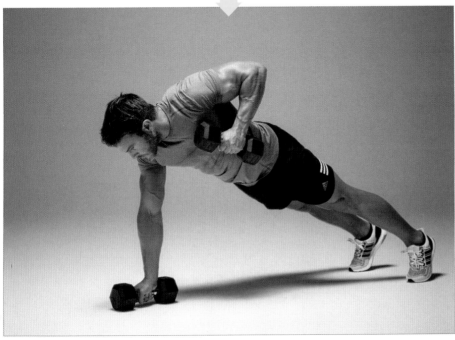

FINISH Row one dumbbell upwards so that your thumb touches your armpit. Lower it back to the floor, then repeat with the other arm. Continue alternating. Try to stay parallel to the floor and don't twist your body.

Dumbbell reverse flye

Target muscles Shoulders, back

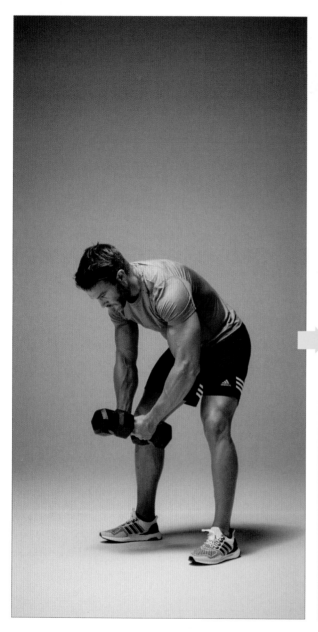 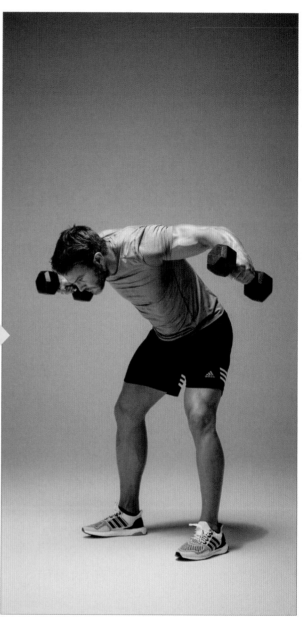

START Lean forwards at the hips with a dumbbell in each hand, with your chest up, core braced and back flat.

FINISH Leading with your elbows, raise the weights upwards as if you were spreading your wings, squeezing your shoulder blades together at the top of the move.

Dumbbell reverse-grip bent-over row

Target muscles **Back, biceps**

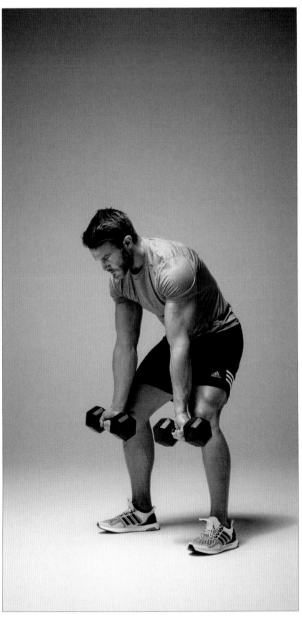

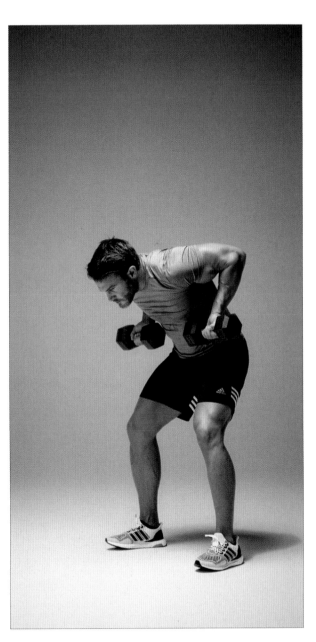

START Stand with your core braced, your back straight and your shoulder blades retracted, holding dumbbells with your palms facing away from you.

FINISH Bend your knees slightly and lean forwards from the hips. Row the dumbbells up, leading with your elbows, until they almost touch your chest. Pause, then lower under control.

Dumbbell shoulder press

Target muscles Shoulders, triceps

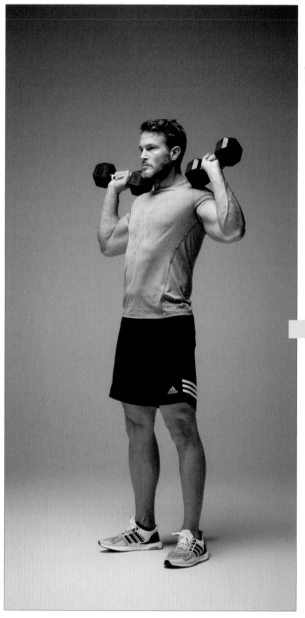 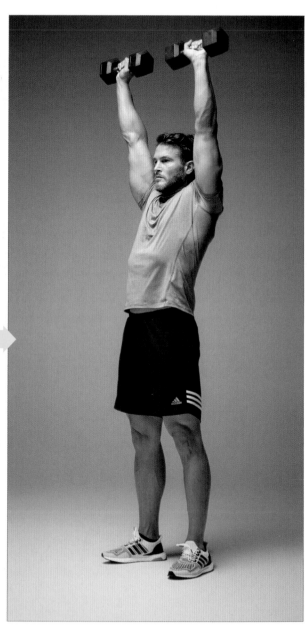

START With your feet shoulder-width apart, hold a dumbbell in each hand at shoulder height with palms facing forwards. Keep your chest upright and your core muscles braced.

FINISH Press the weights directly upwards, keeping your core braced, until your arms are fully extended overhead. Lower back to the start.

Dumbbell side lunge

Target muscles Legs, core

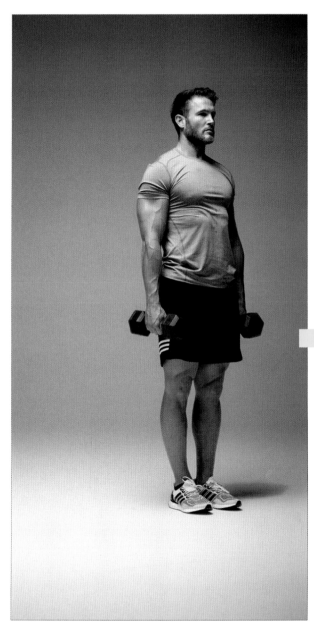

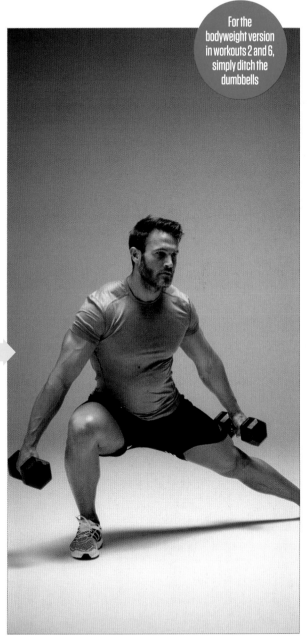

For the bodyweight version in workouts 2 and 6, simply ditch the dumbbells

START Stand tall, holding a dumbbell in each hand with your chest up and core braced.

FINISH Take one step sideways and lower your body until one of your knees is bent at a right angle and you feel a slight stretch in your groin. Push off your foot to reverse the movement. Alternate sides.

Dumbbell split squat

Target muscles Legs, core

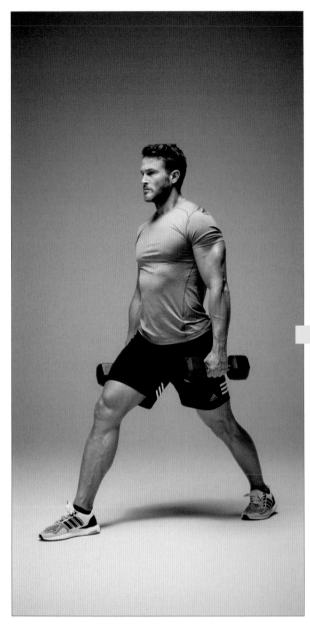

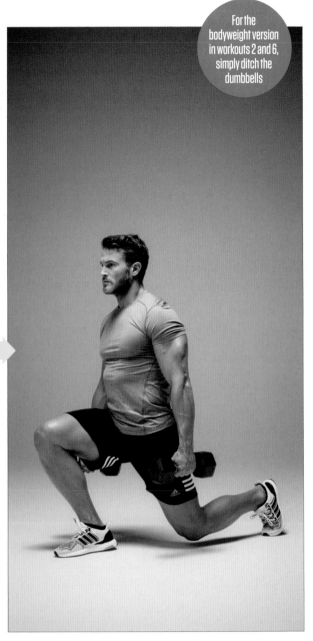

For the bodyweight version in workouts 2 and 6, simply ditch the dumbbells

START Start in a split stance, with one foot in front of the other, holding a dumbbell in each hand.

FINISH Bend both legs until your trailing knee touches the floor. Straighten both legs to return to the start, then go straight into the next rep, alternating sides.

Dumbbell squat

Target muscles Legs, core

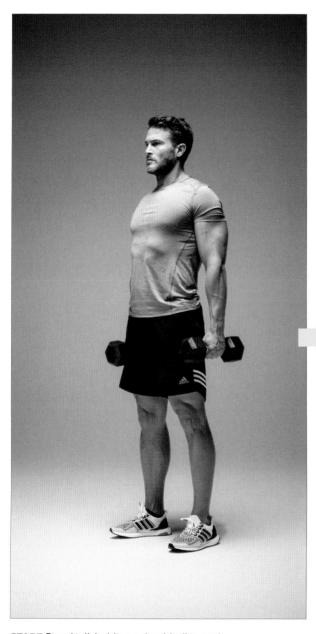

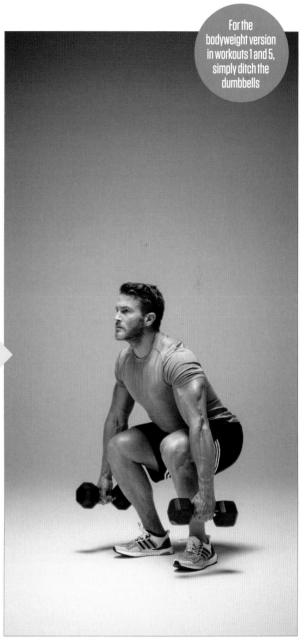

For the bodyweight version in workouts 1 and 5, simply ditch the dumbbells

START Stand tall, holding a dumbbell in each hand with your chest up and core braced.

FINISH Squat down, keeping your chest up, until your hip crease is below the level of your knees. Drive back up through your heels.

Dumbbell squat curl

Target muscles Legs, biceps, core

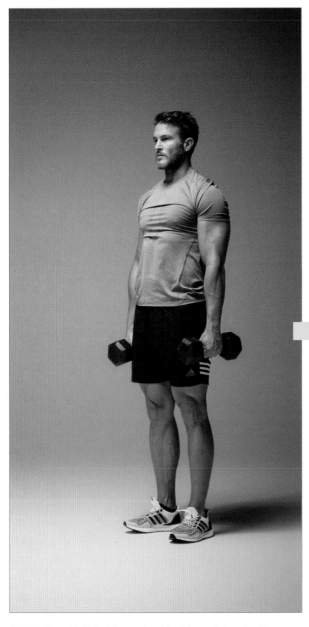

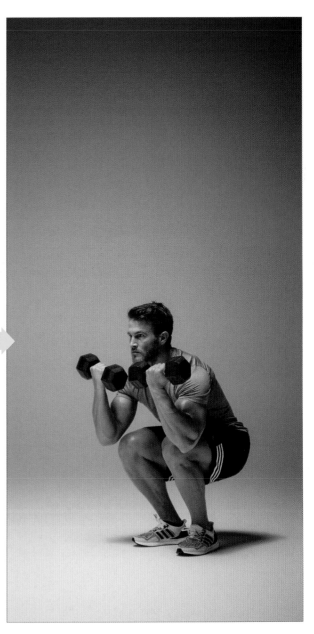

START Stand tall, holding a dumbbell in each hand, with your chest up and core braced. Squat down, keeping your chest up, and at the same time curl the weights up to shoulder height.

FINISH Once your hip crease is below the level of your knees, drive back up through your heels, lowering the weights until your arms are fully straight.

Dumbbell triceps kick-back

Target muscles **Triceps**

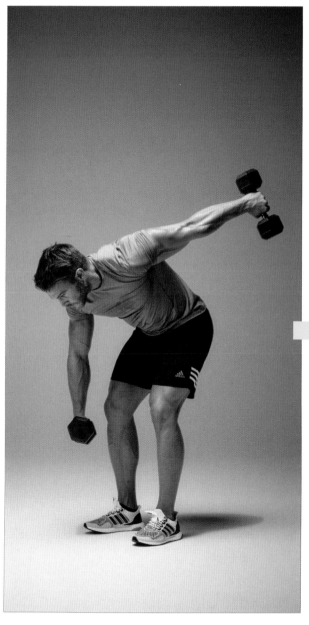

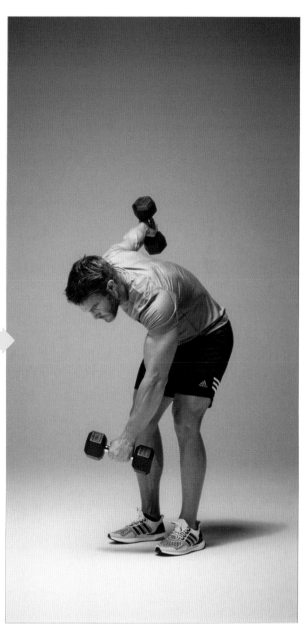

START Holding a dumbbell in each hand, lean forwards from your hips, keeping your back straight and arms bent.

FINISH Raise the weights behind you until your arms are straight, then lower them back to the start.

Dumbbell triceps extension

Target muscles Triceps

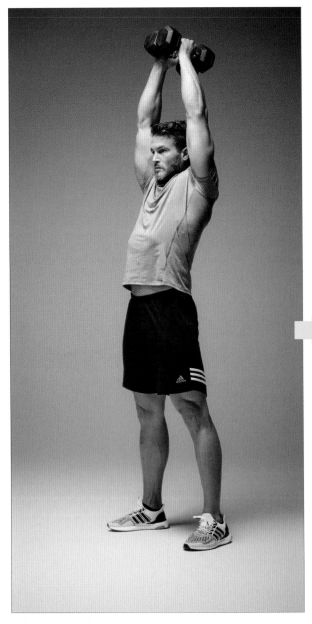

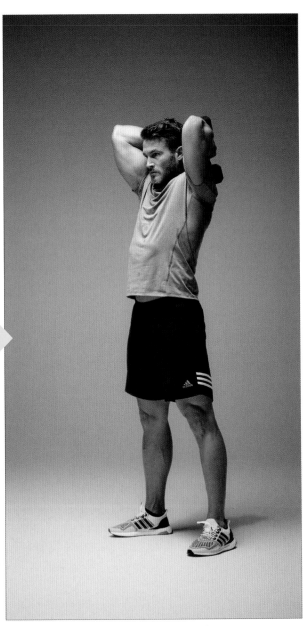

START Stand tall, holding a pair of dumbbells above you with straight arms.

FINISH Slowly lower the dumbbells towards the back of your head by bending your elbows, keeping your upper arms as still as possible. Then raise them slowly back to the start.

Gym ball crunch

Target muscles **Upper abs**

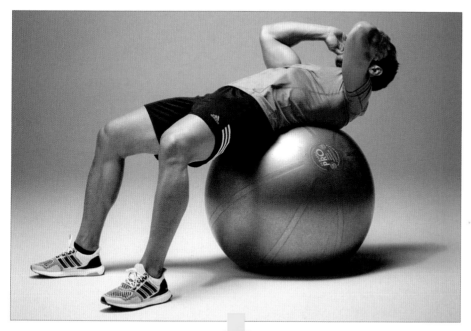

START Lie with your back on a gym ball, your feet flat on the floor and your fingers touching your temples.

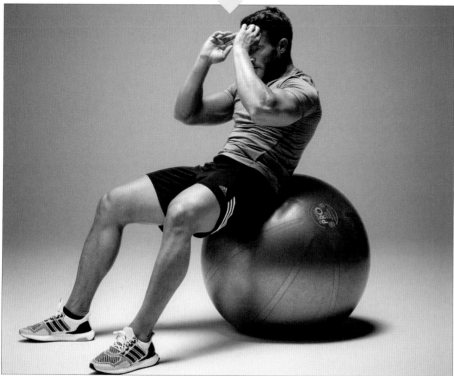

FINISH Contract your upper abs to raise your torso off the ball. Pause at the top, then lower back to the start.

Gym ball crunch twist

Target muscles **Upper abs, obliques**

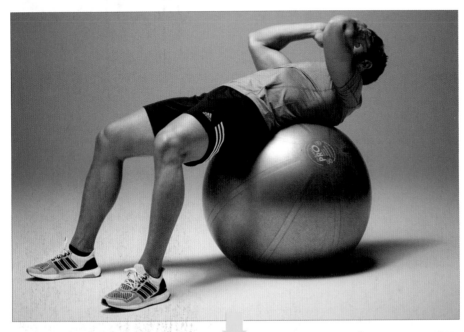

START Lie with your back on a gym ball, your feet flat on the floor and your fingers touching your temples.

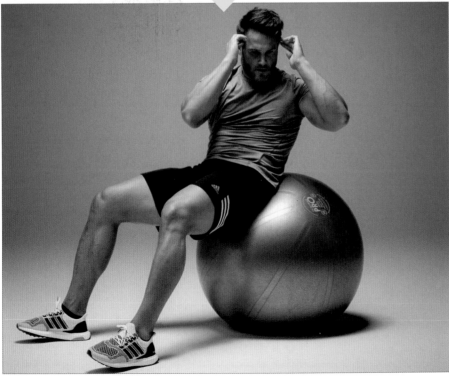

FINISH Contract your upper abs to raise your torso off the ball. As you come up twist to one side, then pause at the top. Lower back to the start then repeat, twisting to the other side.

Gym ball decline plank

Target muscles **Core**

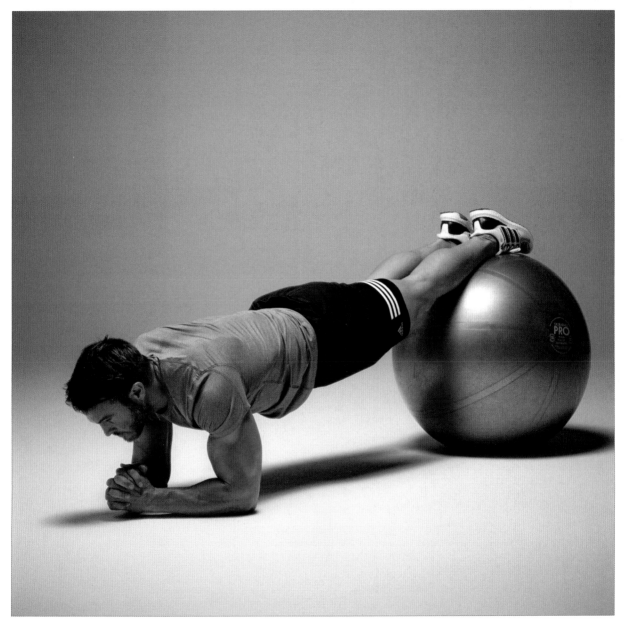

START Get into in the plank position but with your feet on a gym ball.

FINISH Raise your hips to keep your body straight from head to heels.

Gym ball decline press-up

Target muscles Chest, triceps, shoulders, core

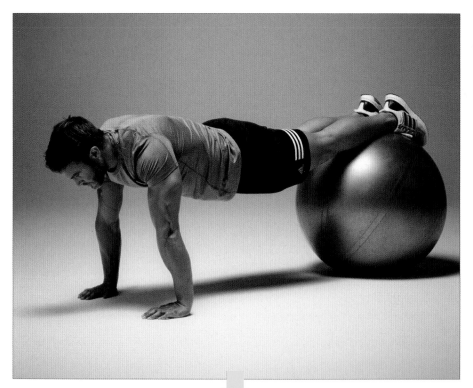

START Get into in the press-up position but with your feet on the gym ball.

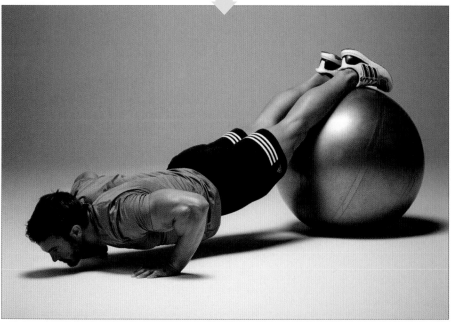

FINISH Keeping your core engaged, bend your elbows to lower your chest to the floor, then press back up to return to the start.

Gym ball dumbbell flye

Target muscles **Chest**

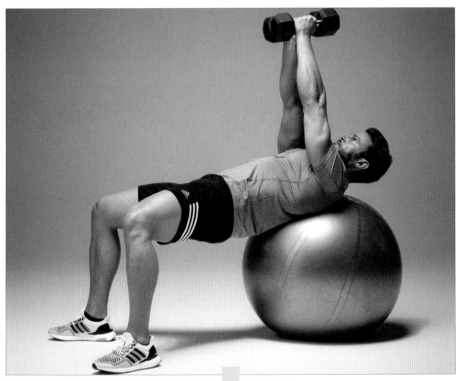

START Lie with your back on a gym ball, your feet flat on the floor and your chest up, holding a dumbbell in each hand in front of your face with arms straight and palms facing.

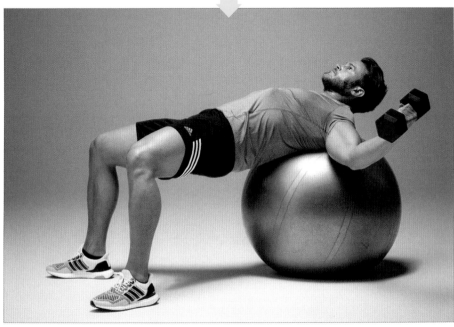

FINISH Keeping a slight bend in your elbows, slowly lower the weights out to the sides until you feel a good stretch across your chest. Then raise the weights back to the start position.

Gym ball dumbbell press

Target muscles **Chest, shoulders, triceps**

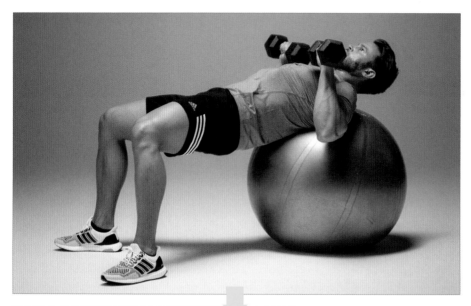

START Lie with your back on a gym ball, your feet flat on the floor and your chest up, holding a dumbbell in each hand by your shoulders.

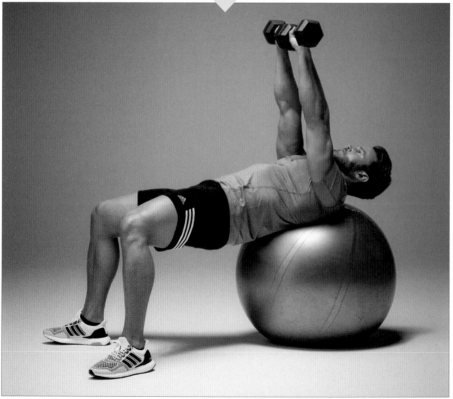

FINISH Press the weights directly overhead until your arms are straight. Then lower them back to the start position.

Gym ball dumbbell pull-over

Target muscles **Chest, back**

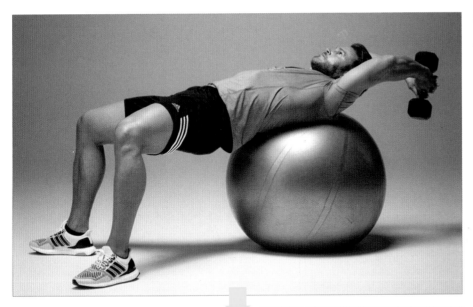

START Lie with your back on a gym ball, your feet flat on the floor and your chest up, holding a dumbbell in both hands directly above your chest.

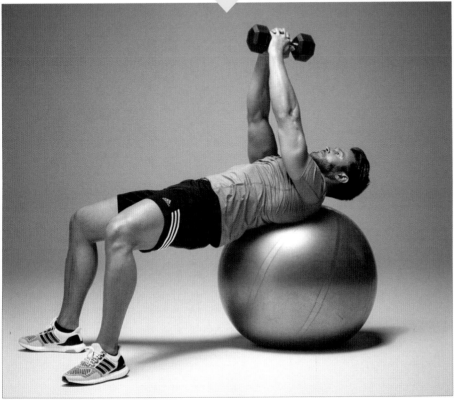

FINISH Slowly lower the weight behind your head until you feel a good stretch in your lats. Then raise the weight back to the start position.

Gym ball incline plank

Target muscles Core

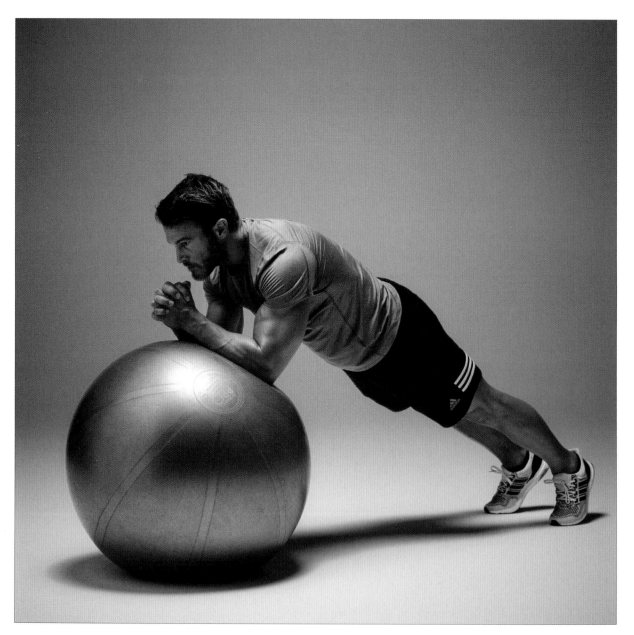

START Get into in the plank position but with your hands clasped together and resting on the gym ball.

FINISH Raise your hips to keep your body straight from head to heels.

Gym ball incline press-up

Target muscles Chest, triceps, shoulders, core

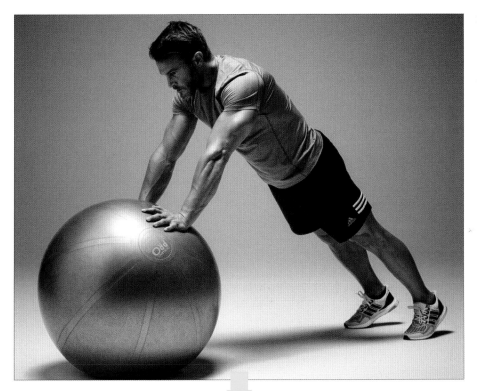

START Start in a press-up position but with your palms resting on the gym ball, hands shoulder-width apart. Brace your core.

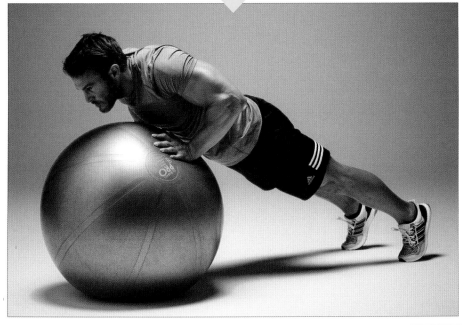

FINISH Bend your elbows to lower your chest to the ball, then press back up powerfully to return to the start.

Leg raise

Target muscles **Lower abs**

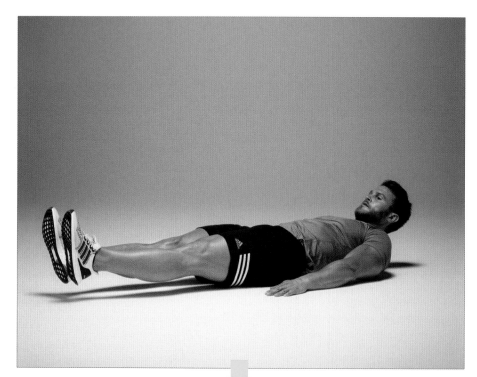

START Lie flat on your back with your arms straight and by your sides and your abs engaged.

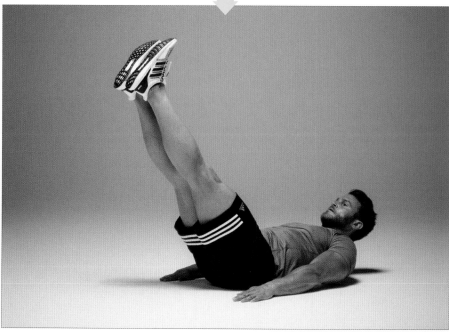

FINISH Keeping your feet together and legs straight, raise your feet as high as you can. Pause at the top, then lower them back to the start under control.

Mountain climber

Target muscles **Abs, core**

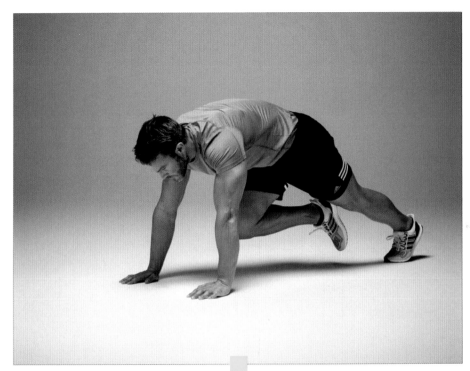

START Start in a position similar to a sprinter on the starting blocks.

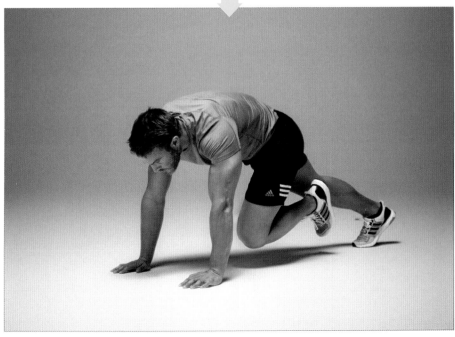

FINISH Bring one knee forwards and across your body, then back to the start. Repeat with the other leg, keeping the movement slow and controlled.

Plank

Target muscles Core

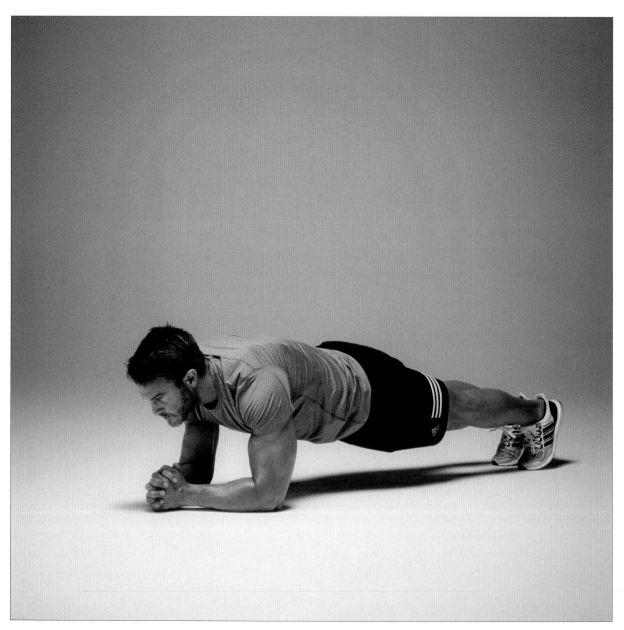

START Get into a press-up position but with your elbows and forearms on the floor and feet close together, keeping your body completely straight.

FINISH Hold the position. To make the move tougher, move your elbows forwards and together.

Press-up

Target muscles Chest, triceps, shoulders, core

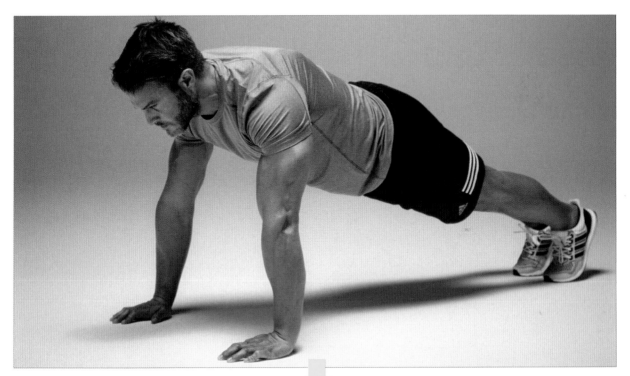

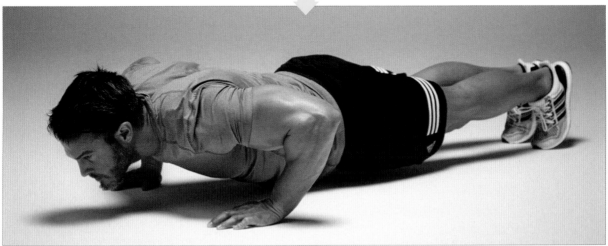

START Get into a press-up position with your hands just outside shoulder width apart. Keep your abs braced.

FINISH Bend your elbows to lower your body until your chest touches the floor – but not your thighs – and then press back up to return to the start.

Reverse crunch

Target muscles Lower abs

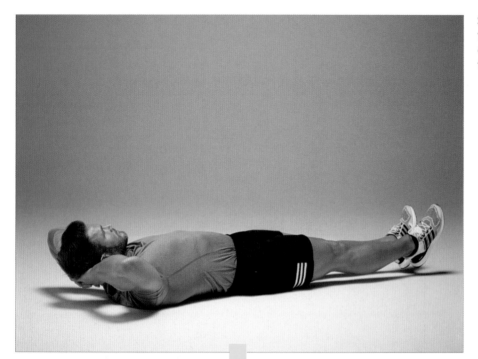

START Lie flat on your back with knees bent and hands either across your chest or touching your temples.

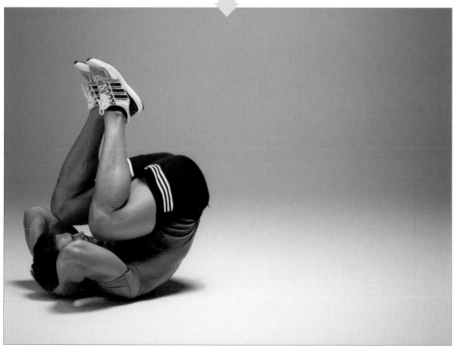

FINISH Contract your abs to lift your shoulders and curl your chest towards your knees. Pause at the top of the move and squeeze your abs, then lower slowly to the start.

Side plank

Target muscles Core, obliques

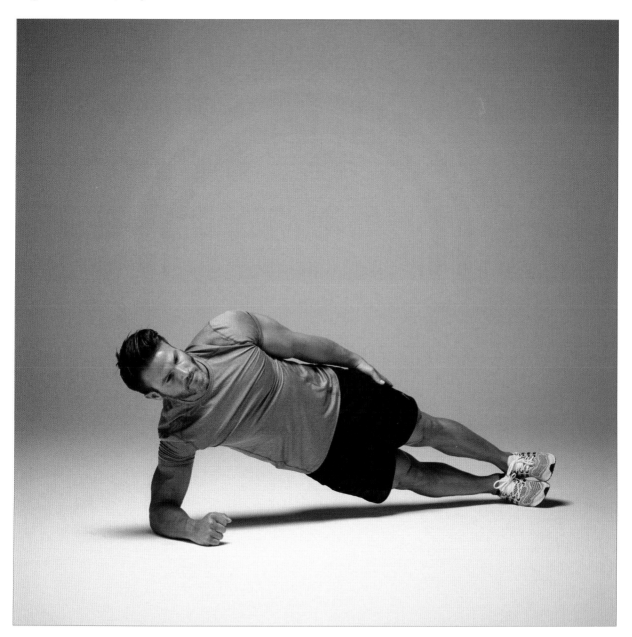

START Get onto one forearm with your feet "stacked" one on top of the other – or both on the floor, one behind the other (known as "staggered") if this is too hard.

FINISH Keep your body in a straight line from head to heels with your core and glutes fully engaged. Hold the position on one side for half the time, then switch to the other side.

Side plank star

Target muscles Core, obliques

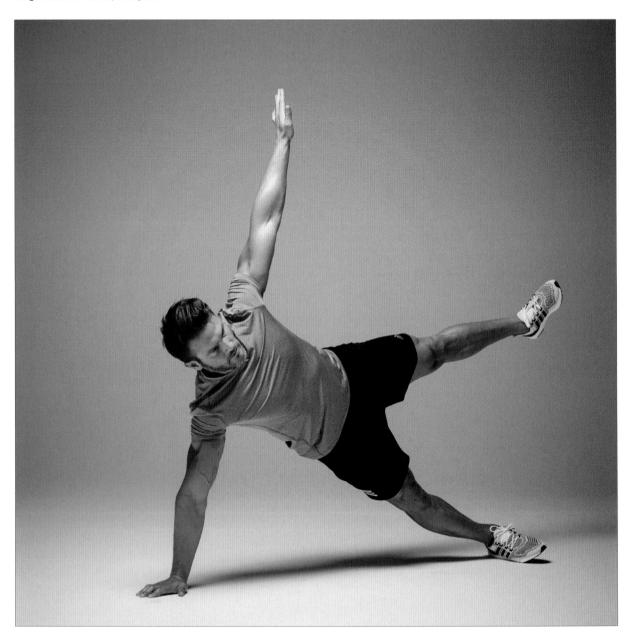

START Lie in a side plank position but rest on your hand instead of your forearm. Your feet need to be stacked.

FINISH Raise your top leg and arm and hold the position. Hold it on one side for half the time, then switch to the other side.

V-sit

Target muscles **Abs, core**

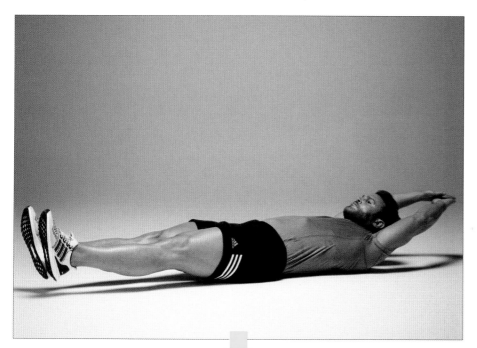

START Lie on your back with your arms and legs out straight. Lift your legs until they're at 45° to the floor.

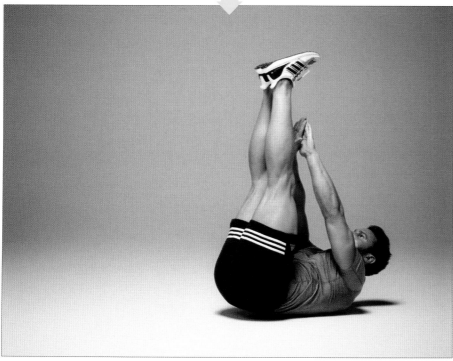

FINISH Raise your upper body to meet your legs, stretching your arms toward your shins. Hold this position for a moment, then go back to the start position.

Wide press-up

Target muscles Chest, shoulders, triceps, core

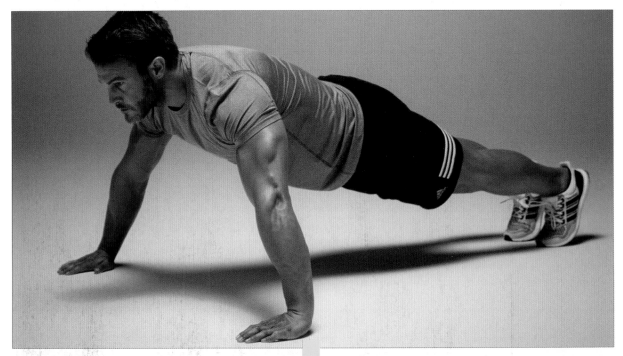

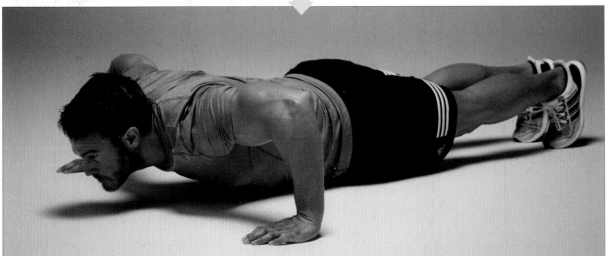

START Get into a press-up position with your hands double shoulder-width apart.

FINISH Keeping your body in a straight line with your abs braced, lower your torso until your chest is just above the floor. Then press back up.